CW00616483

HEALTH P⌐

A THERAPISTS' CONCISE GUIDE
TO ADVERTISING

HEALTH PROMOTION

A THERAPISTS' CONCISE GUIDE TO ADVERTISING

TIM FLANAGAN

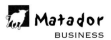
Matador
BUSINESS

Matador
9 De Montfort Mews
Leicester LE1 7FW, UK
Tel: (+44) 116 255 9311 / 9312
Email: books@troubador.co.uk
Web: www.troubador.co.uk/matador

ISBN 978 1906510 442

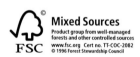

Mixed Sources
Product group from well-managed
forests and other controlled sources
www.fsc.org Cert no. TT-COC-2082
© 1996 Forest Stewardship Council

Typeset in 12pt Book Antiqua by Troubador Publishing Ltd, Leicester, UK
Printed by Cromwell Press Ltd, Trowbridge, Wiltshire, UK

Matador is an imprint of Troubador Publishing Ltd

For Maria, who always loves me and inspires me

Contents

Introduction

Marketing and promotion are not always considered to be relevant to health care professionals who rely mainly on reputation or lack of competition to bring in a steady flow of patients or clients. However, in light of recent awareness of rising obesity levels, the UK has become more health conscious, demanding a quality service 'right here, right now.' With demand comes the need for supply and many complimentary, as well as historically traditional clinics, are becoming common place in our towns and high streets, providing competition to the government managed Health Service.

People often have the perception that if they want a quick and high quality service they will have to pay for it. This willingness to put their own money into their health and well-being creates the basis for a competitive and lucrative market.

However, on its own a positive reputation is no longer enough to keep the clients coming through the door.

Certainly, after you and your clinic are established, your reputation and clients' recommendation of you should maintain a healthy bank balance, but at the start of any business or to expand and grow an already established business, you will need to learn how to market and promote yourself.

The market place is becoming swamped with so many different types of medical services, complimentary therapies and holistic therapies, that it is becoming harder for people to choose the right service they need. It is up to you to promote yourself effectively so that the general public is well educated and informed about what it is you provide. You will then start to get new patients.

As part of your training for your specific profession you will probably have learnt about the theory and history behind your profession, how to treat and manage patients, clinical standards, medical conditions and even developed a dictionary of new words and phrases relating to the professional and medical aspects of your job. Very few health care professionals are actually taught about business. It's not enough to just know about your job and nothing else, you need to know how to run a business and actively promoting yourself is a key element to a successful business.

There is much more to marketing than simply advertising, which is really the end product of market research. Before thinking about how to advertise you will need to understand your market place. This includes your locality, your potential customers and your competitors.

The aim of this book is to make you aware of your clients and tell you how you can attract more. A greater understanding of who you are selling your service to as well as who your competitors are and how their services compare to yours, will provide you with a unique insight into your position in that market place. From this position you can easily gain new clients, whilst guaranteeing existing ones stay with you.

Once you have a grasp of who you are selling your product to you will have a better understanding of how to create effective advertising. Advertising is an exciting part of any business; its intention is to rapidly increase the flow of clients to you. Get it right and you will soon fill up the diary, but if it's wrong it could affect your professional credibility as well as the cash flow of the business. A well crafted piece of advertising or promotion will have benefits for your business a long time after the advert has stopped running. You can also develop brand awareness, where a business becomes so easily identifiable that when a potential client needs a certain product they automatically think of you even if you are not running an advert at that particular time. Creating brand awareness is just as important for health care professionals as it is for any business. If you think of any popular petrol company, fast food retailer or clothing brand, they have all created brand awareness whereby you know about them because you recognise a logo or image which is associated with the product.

You can create this brand awareness yourself, all be it only locally, but you will immediately be the professional which potential clients turn to when they need you.

The ideas and concepts contained within this book can all be used and adapted to suit your profession.

With a bit of research and thought your market research and advertising will form an essential part of your business which should be constantly updated and monitored, and you will also find that your business will develop its own forms of promotion over time.

SECTION A

MARKETING

Marketing

*Identifying your typical buyer for promoting
and selling your product or service to.*

—

1

Understanding your market

As with any business, health care professionals need to understand their customers; who they are, whether there are sufficient numbers of them and whether they have enough money to spend on such services. What you also need to consider is how many other similar services you will be competing against.

This is called Market Research and is vital to help your business grow and become successful, but more importantly to convince any investors in your business that their money is being invested in one which is in the right marketplace. This will give them much more confidence in backing you as they are more likely to see a return on their investment. Market research is not just an exercise which needs to be done at the start of a business to form part of the business plan, but something which should be continually evaluated and changed. Your market will change over time, including your customers and your competitors' services and the only way that you can stay ahead of the competition is to asses your market regularly and adapt to that change.

Even if you do not need any external financial backing to start a new business, or expand an established one, you should still undertake some market research. If you are putting your own money and possibly even your personal assets at risk, you should want to be 110% certain that your money and home are safe.

Market research needn't be an expensive part of the background fabric of your business, a lot of the work you can do yourself for very little cost, just a bit of time and effort. Do not rush your market research. To get a good overview of how your business will be placed takes time and any errors or oversights here will show up in your business later, which could, ultimately cost your business money and delay or prevent expansion.

Although it might seem a bit tedious and tiresome, market research serves many functions, including:

●   It gives you a better understanding of who
    your customers are and what requirements
    they have.

●   It will give you an indication on the
    suitability of your business location.

- It secures investment.

- It provides information on your competitors.

- It can give you an indication on the possible long term success of the business.

- If will help you to target and promote your business without wasting money unnecessarily.

- It will provide information on how to pitch you services and products, including quality and price.

Market research can be broken down into three main areas

1. Your potential customers.

2. Your service or product.

3. Your competitors.

If you can comfortably understand all these areas in depth then you will have an excellent awareness of your market and how to make your business succeed through effective advertising.

1. YOUR POTENTIAL CUSTOMERS

Through your training and understanding of your client base, you will already have some background research on your potential customers. But there are some things which you will need to research, including:

- What type of customer will use your service? You will need to have an idea of a typical customer, including information on:

  - Age.
  - Sex.
  - Affluence.
  - Background.
  - Job.
  - Activities.
  - Social life.
  - What meeting areas, clubs or organisations they belong to.
  - What newspapers they read.
  - Which radio stations they listen to.

- Is your typical customer likely to change? Will the local social conditions and environment have an effect on your client base?

2. YOUR SERVICE OR PRODUCT

You already know what service you want to offer to customers, but consider what they want or expect too.

- Will you tailor a range of services to cater for different types of customers or stick to one service for one type of customer?

- Will you provide flexibility of appointments? For example, will you do evening appointments for business people at a higher cost?

- Will you provide cheaper services for mass bookings held at external premises such as GP practices or other business premises in the form of a staff incentive package?

- Is the location you have chosen suitable, not just for now, but for the future too?

3. YOUR COMPETITORS

As well as looking at your own business, you need to asses those of your competitors. Finding out their strengths and weaknesses will help you understand how best to pitch yourself. Questions you need answering include:

- How long have they been established?

- Do they provide a similar service? Compare services, products, prices and location to your own.

- What is the general feedback and opinion from your existing patients on your competitors?

Once you have an understanding of what sort of information you will need you will then need to start to look for it and begin your research.

2

Undertaking market research

Once you have an understanding of what sort of information you will need, you can then start to look for it. A lot of research you can do yourself, this is called desk research, or you can get a third party to undertake it for you. The market research you are aiming to do does not need to be of a quality fit for publication, it is simply for your own needs and requirements, and so does not need to be too involved or deep.

When deciding on the budget for your market research it is important to put it into perspective in comparison to the product or service you are providing. For most health care professionals a large budget which involves employing market research firms and long periods of field research is not necessary. Sufficient desk research can usually highlight the necessary facts, all it takes is a little of your time. Much of the information you need has already been found and is available if you know where to look. Preliminary market research gives you a better idea and understanding of the sort of information you can ask a research agency to find out on your behalf if you do end up going down that avenue.

There are two types of research:

1.   Quantitative – this is basically to do with statistics, such as '73% of people said they would use a Reflexologist.'

2.   Qualitative – this is more about understanding behaviour, i.e. 'why do people need a Reflexologist?'

To start finding out the information, you will find access to the internet is really useful. If you haven't got a computer with internet access at home, local libraries usually have PCs which can be used free of charge, but you may be limited to 1 hours use per visit.

Overall, most of the information you will need, will only be very locally relevant to you, so you would be wasting your time and energy trying to look up information in areas such as Companies House in London. Companies House is the main source of information on businesses, their finances and directors in the UK. Most businesses start at Companies House to look at similar businesses and what sort of competition they will form, however, many of the businesses you will be competing with for a share of the local market will not be registered at Companies House and those that are, will not be direct competition unless they are operating within a certain radius of where your business is.

You first stop for desk research should be the internet. A lot of relevant information is already available to you free of charge. The internet should be able to give you information on your competition as well as the local area and its residents. Unfortunately it will be very weak on providing information on your customers' opinions, to gain that you are going to have to go out and ask them. This is called field research.

The following websites provide different information and data which you will need to sift through to find what is relevant to your business. There are many types of directories which you can look up on the internet and all provide very similar information about your competitors. Listed here are just a few.

www.yell.com

This is the online version of the Yellow Pages directory and lists information on local businesses that you will be in direct competition with.

When you visit the site, simply add in the service you are intending to provide together with the location you will be working from and click 'Search.' The results are then displayed, sometimes accompanied by other similar businesses in the wider area. Most will simply be a list of names, addresses and telephone numbers; however they may also have links to their websites. The list of businesses featured on yell.com is not necessarily every business which is listed in the paper version of Yellow Pages. Businesses pay additional fees to feature in the online version, so you may not have a complete list of your competition.

What information you can gain:

- Locations and contact details of your competitors.

- Brief summary of your competitors services and facilities.

- Link to your competitors websites where you can gain additional information on their services etc.

www.google.co.uk

On the main google page, click on 'Maps' then 'Find a

Business.' You will then need to input the profession you are looking for in one box and the location in the second box. Click on 'Search Businesses' and a list will appear of the businesses you are searching for, as well as a map showing their location.

What information you can gain:

● Names, addresses and a mapped location of your competitors.

www.thephonebook.bt.com

Click on the 'Business Type' link on the main Home page and enter your profession and the location then click on 'Search.' You will then have a list of similar businesses and their details.

What information you can gain:

● Names and addresses of your competitors.

www.thomsondirectories.com

On the Home page of the online version of the Thomson Directory, you can input the type of business you are looking for followed by the location, then click on 'Search.' The resultant list of names will provide you with a comprehensive idea on the level of competition in your area.

What information you can gain:

● Names, addresses and a mapped location of your competitors.

The following website is also useful in finding out information on your local neighbourhood and consequently what the market you are aiming at is like.

www.statistics.gov.uk

By clicking on the 'Neighbourhood' link you will be taken to a page where you have access to two different types of searches. In the 'Neighbourhood Summary' section enter the postcode of your clinic and click 'Search.' The information which is then displayed is broken down into People, Health, Work, Education, Housing, Crime and Environment. There is also an easy to see summary in the form of a swingometer.

What information you can gain:

● Information on the ages of the population in your area.

- The health of the population of the area in comparison to the country as a whole.

- Percentage of your local population who are in work or retired, and consequently whether they could afford private healthcare.

- And much more.

If you are going to do some field research, where you literally get out of your house and talk to people, you are going to have to work out who it is you need to interview. To do this you need to imagine a stereotypical patient who comes to your clinic. Think about the average age range and whether they are men, women or children or all. This is going to be the start of your criteria for your respondents. Other factors can also be included depending on your profession and what sort of clientele you are looking to appeal to, such as whether they are retired or in full time employment and whether they visit a gymnasium regularly etc. You will then need to think about how many people will be taking part in your field research. Professional agencies will use larger sample numbers than you will probably have access to, but set yourself a reasonable target, maybe 50, so that you can get an idea of whether there are sufficient potential clients in the area, what places they visit, including your competition and any other information which may be relevant to a successful advertising campaign.

Field research can take the form in many ways:

● Talking to people in person.

● Talking to people on the phone.

● Postal Questionnaires.

However you decide to produce a piece of field research, you need to make sure that the questions that people are asked are all the same as well as being in the same order. Sit down and think about what information, both Quantitative and Qualitative that you want to obtain and write it down in a simple form with tick boxes as well as spaces for additional comments. This additional space is very important to obtain Qualitative information allowing people freedom to express the thoughts and reasoning behind their answers.

If you decide to post questionnaires to people be aware that the response rate is usually quite low. To increase the chance of getting a completed questionnaire returned to you, include a stamped addressed envelope, write an accompanying letter or offer a reward or prize for those who respond.

Interviewing on the telephone can be a costly way of accumulating market research and the respondent may not always be relevant to your research. If you are doing face to face interviews make sure the first question you ask ascertains whether or not the respondent fits your criteria.

If you have decided to use an agency to produce your market research, you will have to decide whether or not it is going to be worth the money you pay for it. Because your business is not going to be a large multinational company selling millions of pounds worth of products, a costly market research report from an agency may not be justified compared to the fees you will be collecting from your patients. Most of the time you will gain a good idea of your markets habits by doing your own simple market research.

If however, you still want to use an external agency, you will need to do some preparation of your own before approaching them. This will then enable you to put together a research brief which should outline the purpose of the research, the type of respondent you are aiming for, questions you need answering, what you want from the agency, i.e., advice, data or a report, and the time scale. Some companies may give you a fixed price for their services however; others may charge you for what is required depending on the complexity.

Once you have obtained information by performing market research in any form, you are responsible for all the data collected and there should not be any sales calls generated after the research. All information that respondents give is confidential and they should be made aware of this before they participate. They should also be told that the data and views you are recording will not be given to any third party.

It is wise to register with the Data Protection Agency if you are holding information about people.

3

Writing your market plan

A marketing plan can be just as important as a business plan, but is so often forgotten.

To be able to write a plan, you first need to ask yourself a lot of questions about the business. Your answers will then be the basis for the plan, highlighting strengths and weaknesses and giving a prognosis for growth now and in the future.

The success of your business is not just about how well prepared you are or how high tech your equipment is, but more to do with pitching the right product or service to the right people. If the market for your service does not exists or is already oversubscribed by others providing the same service, then you may need to look elsewhere.

A marketing plan analyses the customers your service will apply to. You will already have a good idea of the type of customer who will use your service, including age, sex, affluence, past times etc. By identifying a type of person and understanding about their lifestyle you gain information on where to advertise and promote yourself. This prevents you spending money needlessly on advertising in inappropriate places. If you are intending to develop or change an aspect of your business, how will the market respond? The site of your clinic within a community will usually restrict your market place to within a few miles around you, so make sure the highest concentration of suitable customers is within this area.

How is that market growing or changing? Does your market change? If people die or move away in large numbers because of external or social factors you have no control over, it will affect your business and your position within the market has changed. Is the market growing? Within most health services, patient care is increasing primarily because people are living longer, so potentially your market is growing. But what about changes to income and Pensions? Will customers always have the financial means to attend private health clinics?

How do you intend to be best placed in that market? How do you intend to be the business that customers turn to when they have a problem? You will need to culture a positive reputation that puts you at the forefront of people's minds whether they have been to you before or not. Think about how you are going to advertise and promote yourself and your practice. Consider the advertising you have already done in the past; does it portray the right image, was it professional, did it actually get any new patients coming through the door? Although we don't always think that brand awareness necessarily applies to health professionals, it is a tool that puts your clinic in potential patients mind for when they require your services. If you have a clinic logo, make sure it is on all literature to do with the clinic including all leaflets, letters and reminders. Make use of the space inside and outside of the clinic, put the logo in a prominent position so that passers by will notice it. When advertising, try to make the advert and logo stand out as much as possible. When providing talks or demonstrations have your logo enlarged and on display. Tunics, sweatshirts and polo shirts with the logo on also work well if providing a demonstration or service outside of the clinic. Even if people don't use your services immediately they are aware of you and know what you provide. This ensures that you are adequately placed in the market to be the first practitioner that patient's think of when they need you.

Why will customers need you? If you can work out the

needs of your patients and what they most regularly want from you, then you can streamline your business to provide the best service. But is there enough room for you in the local market? Do customers need you? Careful analysis of the market place and information on the population local to your practice, together with the level of competition will give you a good idea as to whether your customers need you in the area. If you are already established and the market place changes you are going to have to change with it.

What are your competitors doing? Analysis of your market is not just about your customers. The market will change because of what your competition is also doing. It is a good idea to keep some information on your competitors including their services, prices, availability of appointments, their staffing arrangements, technology and the general opinion from other patients. It is not unethical to phone around your competitors and find out what they are doing. You can be sure that they will be doing it to you. You will also need to estimate the share of the market that they have. This will be based on the time they allocate for treatments, the number of days they work at the clinic, the number of employees they have working for them and the length of time they have been established. Although it's very difficult, try to calculate what your competitor's strengths and weaknesses are, this may give you an idea of what your clinic could provide that is unique to you. Keep your eyes open and make notes on what advertising and promotion they are doing, together with developments they announce.

What makes your business unique? Every business needs to have something which is unique to themselves and in a lot of businesses it will be a product or design, but healthcare providers have to think in a different way. To many of your patients, the most important and unique aspect of your business is you and the service you provide. Offering a better package of care than your competitors will give you the edge you need to gain new patients, but more importantly retain existing ones. Offering a service which is cheaper than your competitors is not necessarily a unique selling point, patients will often put customer care at a higher perceived value to the price they pay. But it's not just about how they are treated inside the clinic, but it is also about the clinic itself. How accessible it is, the comfort of the reception area, friendliness of the staff, cleanliness of the building and what facilities and technology you have, are all aspects of the clinic and your business that will influence whether a patient will come to you. If your business is unique, you are more likely to generate repeat custom as well as generating a positive impression that the patient will convey to their friends.

How do you intend to gain customers? If you've assessed your market correctly, the actual process of advertising and promoting your clinic should be relatively easy. You know who you are targeting, you understand a bit about their lifestyle and what areas and places they visit so all you now have to do is tell these people that you are available. This can be done in many ways from placing an advert into a publication or leaflet that they will receive, or directly promoting your clinic to them in a face to face manner. There are many ways you can promote your clinic for very little money, some for nothing more than a little bit of time and effort. As part of your marketing plan you should clearly state how you intend to advertise your clinic and what you intend your budget for the year to be. Try to estimate the cost of each particular type of advertising you intend to do and what sort of returns you would expect to get back.

Once you have written your plan, get it proof read by two other people, usually family members or colleagues, who may notice errors you hadn't seen, or may point out a section which needs further clarification.

Like a business plan, you should aim to review your marketing plan at least once a year. Many factors will cause you to adjust your plan including professional restrictions, government legislation, your competitors, changes to the local market, the direct costs of providing the service to patients and your advertising budget.

Constantly review the four main key areas for marketing success;

● Service

● Price

● Location

● Customers

By doing this you should be able to maintain a strong position in the market, advertise effectively and for maximum profit and withstand the threat of a smaller market share from competitors.

If you have to present your marketing plan at some stage to a bank or other potential investors, they are not only looking at the potential of the business, whether it ís new or developing; they are also interested in you as a person. They come across many businesses, but what makes it different is if the person behind the plan has the drive, energy and enthusiasm to take it through and succeed. Make sure that you rehearse your presentation, time it and allow for questions. Take visual aids with you to enhance, support or demonstrate what you are intending to do. Be clear but realistic about your aims and how yours compare to your competitors. When responding to questions keep your answers concise and to the point. Do not become defensive if you receive criticism or comments about aspects of the business. Turn the criticism around and work on the flaw it has exposed. Keep eye contact with your audience, speak clearly and try to maintain enthusiasm for the business.

SECTION B

BRANDING

Branding

Create an identifiable image which is only associated with your business.

4

Brand Awareness

By creating an awareness of your business as a brand you will be putting yourself forward to potential customers as their first choice to receive treatment from. If a potential customer already has an idea of the level of service they can expect to receive from you even though they have never been before, then you have created a positive brand. With health care professionals, your brand will usually come in the form of reputation and recommendation from existing clients. But for those potential customers who do not know you or do not know anyone who has already been to see you, creating an awareness of you and your business as a brand is relatively simple and will help you to stand out from the competition.

Developing a brand need not be expensive. The most you will need is some thought, time and effort. There will of course be some expenses in the form of signage for the practice, stationery and advertising, but even the advertising need not be expensive as shown later in the book, merely taking up some of your time. As with all aspects of your business, you will need to decide what sort of budget you are going to allocate to the branding of your business and it is important to try to stick to it as best you can.

To start recognising how to build a brand you will first need to decide what your brand values are. Brand values are the strengths or qualities which make your business better than your competitors and promote your most positive features. The brand values you may write down will be from one perspective; yours, but include brand values which will also be from the perspective of your customers.

For customers, it is not always about the price of the service you are providing, but also to do with the quality of service, availability of appointments, clinic facilities and location. If you can, ask patients what they think of your service and how it compares with others they may have tried. As part of your market research you should already have a reasonable idea of what potential new customers are looking for. Collate all this information to make a list of brand values which match yours and your customers' requirements for your business. If your values vary too much from your customers you may need to reconsider or be flexible enough to provide what customers want. If you don't appeal to enough customers you are not going to have a business which develops quickly with a good reputation or a positive brand image. In short, your business may not relate to its market and consequently fail or at best be a mediocre success.

EXAMPLES OF BRAND VALUES

A Physiotherapist owns a practice which also includes two other Physiotherapists. The following may be listed as the brand values for the business, some of which should be unique to that business.

- Excellent professional skills – Up to date, constantly expanding range of knowledge.

- Availability of appointments – Out of hours as well as Saturday appointments.

- Variety of professionals – Male and female Physiotherapists to suit different customers needs. Larger range of skills and knowledge available to customers.

- Excellent value of money – By comparison to

the competition, the Physiotherapist offers longer appointments at a comparable price.

- Customer care – Practice telephone is constantly manned by a receptionist.

- Modern surgery – Up to date equipment in the surgeries. Clean and modern waiting area with relaxing and comfortable amenities.

- Modern facilities – On line internet booking for appointments for increased customer choice.

- Surgery location – Situated in town high street with parking facilities. Within easy reach of bus route.

- Links with other professionals – Excellent links with a Podiatrist, Sports Masseur, Sports Coach, Rehabilitation Specialist, and Orthopaedic Surgeon to offer a greater overall treatment.

Once you realise what your brand values for your business are you will then need to consider how you are going to communicate them to your potential customers. There are many forms in which this communication can take, different ones picking up on different values but collectively they will inform customers about what sort of service you provide.

Important areas to consider include:

- Your business name and logo.

- Your slogan.

- The appearance of your premises both internal and external.

- The stationery and literature you use or produce.

- The appearance of your staff.

- Where you advertise.

- How your adverts appear.

When considering each form of communication, try to relate it to your brand values as much as possible. Include information on the values wherever you can, especially where there is room for text and information such as the inside and outside of the clinic and on the stationery and literature your patients or other health care professionals will receive. Your business name and slogan, if you have one, need to communicate the brand values whilst not expanding too much on them.

Once the communication of your brand values is in place you will create a strong and lasting image of your business in the minds of your customers, as well as those that have never been to you.

If you work with associates or employ staff, ask them for their input on the branding to see if it conveys the right impression. Make sure all staff are happy to be part of the brand and adhere to the brand values.

EXAMPLE

You have spent a lot of time and effort on your brand values, have modern facilities, continually updated skills and knowledge and spent much of your advertising budget on an advertising campaign. On the telephone, the receptionist sounds bored, uninterested and obstructive, so patients are not booking an appointment to see you and your whole list of brand values is now breaking down. Your brand is now not appearing to be what you were aiming for because the entire thing has been destroyed by the receptionist's poor communication. If you are relying on staff they must also portray the right brand values.

Although brand awareness is important, there is no benefit to be gained by rushing it all at once to get it in place immediately. Take your time over it and think carefully about how you want your business to be perceived. If your budget is restricted, you can always phase business changes in over time; your business will still develop its brand image to customers.

Customer feedback is a great way to know if you are delivering on the values that you are putting forward. You can do this verbally by simply asking the patients or by sending a letter to them after the appointment. This is also a good way of developing good customer relations so that they talk about you to their friends and create free word of mouth advertising.

As part of your market research you will have already found and understood what it is that your customers want or need. Unfortunately those needs change over time and you will need to re evaluate them and therefore adjust your brand to keep it in line with your customers requirements otherwise you could run the risk of being left behind.

5

Choosing a Name for Your Business

When you start a business and write a business plan, a lot of emphasis is placed on finances, premises, staff, equipment and many other areas of a new business, but very little thought goes on the name of the business. In some ways, this is the most important aspect of the 'image' of the business you could possible choose, but most of the time it is hastily thought up or simply named after you, the practitioner.

Using your own name as your business name is perfectly alright and works very effectively if someone is looking for you by name in the telephone directory, especially if they have been recommended to come and see you. But what about those clients who haven't heard of your name before? Your personal name does not describe what profession you provide unless it is followed by the name of your profession. For example, if a client sees the name 'Andrew Smith,' they won't realise that he is an Osteopath. But simply putting the profession after the name explains a lot more. 'Andrew Smith, Osteopath' works on two levels, it links the name with the profession so the client knows what it is they do, but also introduces the client to a friendly know contact which hopefully they will remember and forever associate with the profession when they need to use it. Be careful about using letters of qualification after names as part of the business name, because most of the time they won't be of great relevance to the general public. Of course, they need to be told you are appropriately qualified, but this can be done in other ways.

Even an existing business would do well to look at their name and make changes if necessary. Renaming could change your business overnight and could be the simplest way of generating brand awareness and gaining new clients.

Look at your business name, what does it say about you? Is it professional? Does it convey the right image? Is it memorable? Does it say what it needs to say?

Before any potential clients even contact you, they will be influenced by and form an opinion of you and your service based on the name of your business. Choosing the right name is the start of developing a brand which clients will always associate with you and the exceptional service you provide. Coupling a name with a logo can enhance brand awareness of you even more; a picture is instantly more recognisable than words.

Sometimes obscure and abstract names seem to work well. Using a totally unrelated word or name provides a blank canvas onto which you can imprint and culture an image which only relates you to that name. You don't have to look far to see products or businesses whose names have nothing at all to do with describing their service, but you will automatically associate the name with the company.

Try to avoid the temptation of calling yourself a name beginning with the letter 'A' just for the sake of being the first in the listing in telephone directories. It will probably be a totally irrelevant and meaningless name and if someone else is doing the same it appears to be competitive and unprofessional.

Choosing a suitable name can be done for you by professional firms who would come up with a good name, but at a cost. This could be quite large and not at all proportionate to the volume of income your business will generate, so may not be an appropriate option. Instead, you can easily do it yourself by following the guidelines set out here.

To start with make a descriptive and concise list of all the words and phrases which describe your job as well as words associated with your profession. You might want to enrol the help of a friend or family member to help you; their opinion is vital. Keep each one limited to a maximum of three words. Now think about your clients and cross out all the words that they either won't understand or won't realise the relevance of it to you. Looking at your competitors, cross out names which look or sound similar to theirs. Think about each name carefully and separately and try to interpret what feelings, impression and description each one conveys to you. Cross out all that are not right. Look at the check list below and condense your list to about 5 names. Once you have these, you could always perform a small bit of market research on your family and friends to gain their opinions and see if your name conveys the image you want. You might then be down to around 3 names of which you could choose the most popular or simply select the one you yourself like best of all. Sometimes, it is a good idea to put the list of names away for a couple of weeks then return to them. Looking at them with fresh eyes may make the final decision clearer. Performing a dummy run of the name on stationery may give you a different view on how each name will actually look in situ.

Ideas for creating a suitable name:

● Be original.

● Make it recognisable.

● Make it simple and snappy.

● Ensure it reflects your business and communicates the image of the business.

● Make sure you like it, after all you have to live with it.

● Link the name to the area where you work. Clients will automatically link with the area and feel that you are a local and friendly professional. Because your catchment area is going to be restricted to the local area and not national, you won't have to worry about changing the name at a later stage to reflect something bigger than just the town, city or county you work in.

● Include humour or play on words but keep to the   point and avoid cheesy and corny lines and phrases otherwise you will be remembered for all the wrong reasons.

- Make the name meaningful.

- Make sure it is easily pronounceable. Clients will avoid saying your name if they cannot pronounce it and word of mouth advertising will be effected.

Things to avoid:

- Offensive words or expressions.

- Do not include the words British, Scottish, National or International without permission.

- You are not allowed to use the words Charity or Trust unless you actually are registered as a charity.

- Unauthorised use of professional titles.

- Appearing to give the impression that your business is connected to the government or royal family.

- Avoid embarrassing names that, if spelt differently could portray the wrong impression.

- Try to avoid merging two words together.

- Discard boring and unimaginative words.

- Avoid names that are too obscure and have no meaning.

Once you have chosen what you are going to call your business, it is wise to check that no one has used the name before you print any stationery or signage. Go to the Companies House website at www.checksure.biz and input the name into the Company Search section and click on Search. This website lists companies and not sole traders, so also check local business directories and run a search on the internet for any sole traders who may be using the name. If a sole trader is using the same name but does not work anywhere near you, you should be safe to use it too. However, you also need to be careful to avoid names or even similar names which are registered as a Trademark. Check at www.ipo.gov.uk/tm.

If you trade as a limited company, your business name must end with 'Limited' or 'Ltd.' and will need to be registered with Companies House. Sole traders are not allowed to use Ltd or plc after their names

Choosing the right name for your business could be

one of the most important decisions you make. It will not only bring in new clients but keep you ahead of your competitors by keeping your image and brand in front of the public.

6

Designing a Logo and Slogan

The use of a logo as part of your brand image can be quite a powerful tool. It gives a quick recognisable image that customers and potential customers will associate with you and your business and will automatically link in their mind the relationship between the logo and your brand values.

The logo which you choose needs to be:

●   Reproducible.

●   Original.

●   Uncomplicated and clear.

●   Easily recognisable even when reproduced in miniature.

●   Limited use of colours.

- Must not be similar to a logo already in use.

- Must not contain or be part of a copyrighted or trademark image of another company or person.
- If you are using a logo or image that someone else has designed you will need written permission.

Using a limited palette of colours is important for several reasons:

- It appears uncluttered.

- It reproduces easily even when reduced in size.

- It is less costly to print on stationery and literature.

When you look around at well known household company logos, you will see that many of them will only use one colour, which is often the same as the colour of the text making up the business name. Those businesses that do use more colours tend to stick with two or three at the most. Too much colour detracts from the logo itself, keeping it simple and clear helps to make the image instantly more memorable for your customers.

A logo can be used to represent a specific aspect or relationship to part of your business, such as a moving body for a Physiotherapist, a spinal cord for a Chiropractor or a foot for a Reflexologist. But your image needs to be original and chances are that these easily recognisable images are used by numerous health care professionals across the country. This doesn't mean you can't use them, it actually confirms that these are simple and historically successful images that the general public associate with those professions. If you are going to use an easily associated image such as these, sit down with a pen and paper and capture the image in as simple a design as you can, consisting of only a few lines if necessary. What you will then be creating is an original portrayal of this image which customers can instantly link to a profession and to your business.

Logos also give you the freedom to introduce a new image to the public which may be totally unrecognis-able or unrelated to your profession, but inspires conversation and discussion. This also generates word of mouth advertising of you and your business. Many potential customers may also want to come to your practice merely out of curiosity. But be careful, if the image is totally abstract and bazaar people may actually take a dislike to it and therefore be less tempted to use you when they need your services.

Sometimes a logo can be a simple pencil drawing of the practice or premises you work from. This is quite a good way of getting the general public to recognise an actual building and is something tangible which they can remember. Sketches of the practice also look really good on Stationery and portray a highly professional appearance.

You may be tempted to use a logo which consists of the initial letters that make up the business name. These letters can then be reproduced within a circle or square, merged together or used in many other variations to produce a simple logo. Sometimes it is useful to try the initials on the computer and scroll through all the different fonts to find a few that you like but which still project the correct image.

When you have a few different possible logos, get several friends and family members to look at them and give their opinion. It might also help to put the logos away for a few weeks then go back to them with fresh eyes. If you become too absorbed in them during their conception you can sometimes make the wrong decision. Stepping away for a while may give you a fresh outlook on them and give you a clearer idea on which one may be most suitable.

Once you have a logo that you are happy with, it is

important to get it out to the general public and start to make them aware of it. Make sure it is prominently displayed on any signage inside and outside of the practice, all literature, stationery, appointment cards and adverts, bags that contain purchased items, uniform and name badges. Only by displaying it on everything associated with you will your customers link it to you and your business. Customers who don't currently use your services will also become more aware of you through your logo and are likely to recall it at the time they need it. Hopefully, they will also be more likely to phone you if they are looking in the telephone directory and see an image or logo that they already recognise.

SLOGANS

Communicate more to your customers by linking a slogan with your logo on all advertising. Whilst the logo acts as the sign for you and your business, the slogan gives customers a small piece of written infor-mation.

A slogan can be in the form of many things, each of which communicates different messages;

●   Projecting a brand value. If a brand value is

high customer care, a slogan could be 'Patient care is our passion' or 'Taking patient care to another level.' A brand value which demands flexibility and availability of patient appointments could be communicated by the following slogan; 'We're here whenever you need us.'

- Explaining a business goal. If the goal of the business is to provide a continually improving service you could use; 'Striving to provide excellence in back care', 'Providing excellence in Osteopathy' or 'Continually striving to exceed your expectations.' An aim of the business may be to improve accessibility or availability of your health care service to the local community. A slogan could be; 'Bringing Reflexology direct to your home.'

- Describing a benefit of the business to the customer. What would a patient gain from treatment by you? Possible slogans may include; 'Keeping your feet in walking order', 'Your health and fitness comes first,' or 'Massage the stress away.'

The list of slogans can sometimes appear endless, but

as you start to write them down you will gradually get a feel for what you want to say and end up deleting or adapting them as you go. There is no such thing as a right or wrong slogan, but you must feel comfortable with it yourself because, like the business name, you are the one who will have to live with it. As with many business decisions concerning image, talk to family and friends and ask their opinion.

When deciding on a slogan, go back to the brand values you wrote down in preparation for brand awareness and pick out words or phrases that are important to customers and portray a snippet of information about the business. It will need to be a single sentence that is short enough to communicate a message whilst still being snappy and fresh and easily reproducible on literature. Try to avoid corny slogans that will result in more of a groan from customers that pleasurable recognition.

Don't forget to keep you slogan within the boundaries of Advertising Standards (see chapter 7). The same applies to slogans as it does to adverts and no false claims or inappropriate comments should be used.

SECTION C

ADVERTISING

Advertising

*Draw attention to a service usually by announcement
in written, visual or vocal means.*

7

Advertising Standards

Whenever you do any advertising for your business you must be sure that it complies with a set of rules and regulations set by the Advertising Standards Authority.

The legal requirements for your advert are:

- The goods you are selling must match the description of them. (Sales of Goods Act 1979)

- You cannot make your advert misleading or make unfair comparisons with identifiable competitors.

- Do not use a false or misleading description of your goods. (Trades Description Act 1968)

- Your advert must not be libellous, be indecent or contain images which are copyrighted.

- If the marketing communication includes a telephone number such as a mobile phone, charged at a higher than standard national rate, that should be stated.

- If the advert contains a promotional offer, the closing date must be stated, together with your address for the consumer to retain.

- When quoting prices of services or products in an advert, they must be inclusive of all taxes and VAT.

- Your advert should be socially responsible.

- It should not offend or cause fear or distress to the audience without good reason.

- It must not show unsafe, antisocial behaviour or encourage people to break the law.

Non broadcasted adverts are subject to the British code of Advertising, Sales Promotion and Direct Marketing. When broadcasting on television or radio, the codes of practice are enforced by the Committee of Advertising Practice (CAP) Broadcast Committee on behalf of Ofcom.

The guidelines mentioned above apply to the following forms of non-broadcast advertisements:

- Those in newspapers and magazines or in other printed forms.

- Posters in a public place.

- The Internet.

- Sales promotions.

- Direct mail shots.

In all cases you need to ensure that your advert is lawful, but also whether it is morally right; will it cause unnecessary offence or distress?

As well as legal codes for advertising there are also those set by your professional body which may restrict where and how you advertise. It is advisable to check with your professional body and obtain an up to date copy of their guidelines before proceeding with any costly advertising.

If a complaint regarding your advertising is made to the Advertising Standards Authority (ASA) the consequences may include;

- Refusal of further advertising space.

- Bad publicity.

- Costly legal proceedings.

Complaints made by you about one of your competitors or vice versa should first be addressed through your relevant professional body before approaching the ASA.

8

Designing an Advert

Although it may seem to be a perfectly simple and straightforward thing to do, designing an advert that is effective and gets maximum results is a skilled task.

When considering your adverts you will need to monitor all the results from each one so you can continually improve the effectiveness of them. This development towards a tried and tested advert which repetitively gives consistently positive results should follow three main steps.

1. *Testing.* To start with, try many different styles and types of adverts to see which ones generate the highest response of new patients to your business. Also vary which media you use.

2. *Developing.* As you start to find which

adverts work best in different media, start to refine and develop those adverts by changing the odd word, layout or illustration.

3.   *Learning*. Learn what works for different media and why. If a new advertising opportunity arises in the future, you will then have a preconceived idea of which advert would work in that new situation.

This obviously takes time and money to work your way through many different adverts, so why not save a little by doing the testing on yourself and your friends and family. Although it will not accurately represent the general public, it will give you a head start and an idea on how different adverts work. Start by making up many different styles and sizes of adverts, cutting them out and sticking them into a newspaper to see if it grabs your attention when flicking through. You will soon see that certain adverts look better than others. Do some research on costing by contacting the salesperson at the medium you are looking to advertise in and ask prices for different size adverts in colour or back and white, as well as the circulation of the particular publication. You will then need to calculate the number of new patients you would need to attract to recoup the cost of the advert, by assuming they only visit you once. To gain enough new patients so that the advert appears to cost you the same as you have gained in income, is acceptable. To exceed the cost is excellent. Over time those patients may return for more treatment or recommend a friend to you, so the actual long term return on the advertising investment is usually much greater than the initial response. Don't forget that any advertising, no matter how successful it is, is always increasing your profile and the awareness of you in your local community, so none of it is detrimental.

When testing your adverts, don't forget to vary the position of the advert in the media. For example, an advert on the front page of a magazine is much more likely to get better results than one anywhere else in the magazine. It may also be more effective to have an advert alongside an article or feature about some health issue that the magazine has written. The best position in newspapers seem to be on pages 2, 3 and the back page whilst in magazines pages, 1, 3, and 5 tend to work best. Try to arrange for your adverts to be placed near the top of the page rather than the less glanced bottom of the page. Keep a portfolio of different adverts you have used, together with as much informa- tion on it as possible, including the media type, cost, circulation, position and size. It may also be easier to track different adverts by assigning them a specific number or code. When patients contact your clinic and book an appointment you should make a note of where they came from. The easiest way is to get them to bring the advert with them so that they can claim a free gift or discount at the time of the appointment. You will then build up a tally of which adverts work best and bring in the most custom.

HEADLINES

The headline is the most important part of any advert. It is the first thing that readers will look at, even before the illustration, and automatically decide whether or not they are interested enough to continue to read the rest of the information. Don't forget that your advert is directly competing for the readers' time and attention against not only all the other adverts, but the news headlines or articles also in that publication. Put most of your creativeness and energy into designing a good headline, because without it, the copy will not get read no matter how good it is or what amazing offer your have. Of course, you can only write good adverts if you understand the service you are offering and who that service appeals to. Always bear in mind what it is your patients actually want from you and try to get it across in your headline. When considering the best way to get your advert to appeal to as many people as possible, you need to forget why you are advertising and what it is that you, the practitioner, want to gain by it. Instead, put yourself in the shoes of your patient and think about what it is that they want from you and what would appeal to them. Obviously they are mainly looking for treatment but their main objective is the outcome of the treatment, i.e. less or no pain, better mobility, reduced stress, inner calm etc. Other concepts which appeal to patients are treatments at a reduced price, increased speed to get an appointment, high tech facilities, and advancements in the profession. Using this patient appeal in the headline of your advertisements can have powerful affects on the volume of responses it generates.

A headline that works the best is one which is offering a benefit from the reader that only you can provide.

FOOT PAIN GONE OR YOUR MONEY BACK

AROMATHERAPY TREATMENT AT HALF PRICE

HOW TO IMPROVE YOUR BACK IN 30 MINUTES

REDUCE STRESS IN 5 EASY STEPS

Headlines like these grab the attention of those who your advert is relevant to and makes them an offer they can't resist.

News headlines help to gain attention by telling readers about new developments or facts relating to you.

NEW STYLE INSOLES FOR FOOT PAIN

INTRODUCING AN EFFECTIVE TREATMENT FOR BACK ACHE

ANNOUNCING. A PILATES COURSE FOR THOSE WHO WANT TO HAVE NO BACK PAIN

Using headlines that ask a question can often work well, making the reader pause to answer it or arouse curiosity to read the copy to see what the answer is.

DO YOU SUFFER FROM THESE PROBLEMS?

DO YOU MAKE THESE MISTAKES WHEN LOOKING AFTER YOUR FEET?

WHY DO YOUR FEET HURT?

WHATS WRONG WITH THIS SPINE?

These simple headlines basically ask the reader to check with the information held in the copy to see if they can relate to the problems or mistakes listed.

When trying to think up suitable headlines, remember to try and keep the message positive, otherwise all you are doing is portraying an unhappy and uninspiring advert.

All of these headlines use several words to express an idea, concept or offer, but as a small business you may not have the advertising budget to allow you the size of advert which would entertain so many words. Short words and phrases can still work very well for you as long as you keep them punchy and to the point.

One word headlines such as the following ones, can all work quite well, especially the profession titles. If someone has a joint problem and they instantly see the word Osteopathy in large bold letters standing out from the page of their newspaper, they are much more likely to contact the telephone number in the advert.

AROMATHERAPY	MASSAGE
OSTEOPATHY	STRESS
PAIN	ACUPUNCTURE
CORNS	HYPNOTHERAPY

Sometimes using a combination of 2 or 3 words can also be very effective.

FOOT PAIN	MASSAGE AWAY STRESS
BACK ACHE	REFLEXOLOGY FOR £15
REDUCE STRESS	PAINFUL FEET?
STRESS FREE	FREE PHYSIOTHERAPY

A headline does not need to be clever, it just needs to get the readers attention, even if it ties well with the copy within the advert, the reader is unlikely to have got that far.

Place the logotype, i.e., your logo, business name and address, at the bottom of the advert. After reading the headline, the reader then scans down the advert to see who the advert relates to, thus reading the copy.

When writing a headline, try to come up with as many different ones as possible before cutting it down to a select few. This list should then be adapted by maybe adding or changing words to make the headline more specific or effective.

Emphasise certain words in your headline by making them bolder or bigger than the rest of the surrounding words. The headline:

IMPROVE YOUR POSTURE IN 60 MINUTES
OR YOUR MONEY BACK

could be enhanced by changing the layout slightly and making some words bolder, grabbing the attention of the reader a lot quicker, stopping them as they scan the publication and inspiring them to find out more.

IMPROVE YOUR POSTURE
IN 60 MINUTES
OR YOUR MONEY BACK

Sometimes it works well to start a headline with one of the following words to have instant affect:

INTRODUCING	ANNOUNCING
NEW	NOW
AT LAST	FREE
HOW TO	HOW
WHY	WHICH
WANTED	THIS
BECAUSE	IF

When thinking about the size and style of the font you use in your adverts you need to consider what is the clearest and most eye catching. Try not to use fancy artistic text as it will not grab the attention of the reader as they scan through the newspaper or magazine. Don't forget that you are trying to get a message across and generate sales, not win a design or art contest.

Your headline will need to be large and bold in comparison to the rest of the text on the page. With long headlines, highlight the important, striking words in larger or bolder text to the rest of the type. Don't mix and match too many different types of font in the same advert.

COPY

The most important part of the copy is the beginning and inparticular the first sentence. It has got to keep the readers attention now that the headline has made them pause with a thirst to know more.

When you sit down to think about what to write, try not to think too hard, but write down everything and anything that comes into your brain. You will probably not use the vast majority of it, but once you've started writing and the ideas are coming, inside all of the text will be the best way to express and deliver the meaning of the advert.

You can go back over all the ideas you have written at a later stage when you can look at it with fresh eyes and a clear head. What you are doing is simply editing what you have written and putting your message across in a clear, concise and effective way.

If your advert allows you space to contain copy, you have the difficult task of getting across the information you want to give in an enthusiastic way.

To write the rest of the copy, think about what information and answers the patient would want to know.

- What does the treatment involve?

- How effective is it?

- What does it cost?

- Where is the clinic?

- Who are you?

By answering these questions and including them in your advert you are part of the way along the process of getting them through the door. Don't waste space in your advert with flowery descriptions or unnecessary text, stick to the facts, that's what will appeal to your readers. By starting your copy in this way, it is a natural progression from the theme you expressed in your headline. If you calm things down in the first paragraph you will loose the interest of the reader and all the thought you put into the headline will be wasted.

Use subheadings in your copy to give people who are scanning through the advert all the relevant information. They are then more likely to see something that is relevant and of interest to them to make them stop and read the copy in more detail.

Keep the language and style of writing in your advert simple. It's quicker and easier to read and understand for the patient and is less likely to alienate them or make them feel stupid. Keep the sentences short and to the point and avoid using contractions such as 'We're', 'It's' and 'You'll' instead of 'We are', 'It is' and 'You will.'

If you include some illustration, make sure you use a caption underneath it to enhance its importance and meaning. Captions act like subheadings and often stand out against the copy and are more likely to be read first. It may seem obvious, but any pictures and illustrations should be directly relevant to the service or product you are selling, otherwise it won't make any sense to your audience.

The best result you can expect from any advert is to get an immediate response and have the diary full. But you need to encourage this quick response from the reader otherwise their interest will falter and they will put off, or delay, making an appointment with you. In your advert you need to tell the reader what it is they need to do and when. Make any offers date sensitive, i.e. they can only use them for a certain period of time.

If you are using an offer or voucher, vary what it is you are giving away and monitor the results each one produces, even if the headline, copy and publication remain the same. The best responses are undoubtedly always the money off incentives, but try others such as free products. Think about what the patient really wants and what will instantly appeal to them.

ILLUSTRATIONS

If you have room in your advert for a picture, it is wise to have one which relates to the service you are selling, otherwise the wrong sort of reader may stop at your advert and find it irrelevant to them, whilst the reader you are trying to attract has bypassed it altogether.

Consider what type of picture you use. The following will appeal to people your service is aimed at:

● A picture of you in the process of treating a patient

● A picture of the benefits from treatment

● Simple, diagrammatic medical pictures

A photograph tends to work better than an illustration simply because they are much more easily recognised and believable. If a potential patient for example, can see a photograph of you physically treating an existing patient they know exactly what it is they will be getting, rather than an illustration which could be misleading.

If you can use a photograph which has faces and heads on, it is much more likely to stop someone scanning through a newspaper. Faces can also express emotions and thoughts, so if the face of the patient in the above example is showing gratitude and relief from pain, it is much more effective than simple writing it in your copy. If you are using testimonials (see chapter 21) in your adverts, literature or website, a picture of the person who gave the testimonial gives a lot more credibility and believability to that testimonial.

SMALL ADVERTS

When considering your advertising and the budget you have, you will need to decide what size of advert you can afford and this in turn will dictate the possibility of whether or not you use a picture in it. Some adverts still work very successfully even without any pictures and there are ways of securing a good response from small adverts with no pictures.

Small adverts don't normally tend to be in colour and if they do, they can get a bit muddled. Sticking to a single colour such as black or blue and white is the most effective. Because small adverts cost less than full page colour spreads, you can try many different types of adverts to test them and see which get you the best results. You can also run several different adverts in the same publication at the same time highlighting different aspects of the service you provide in the practice. Repeatable adverts increase awareness of your business much more effectively than a single advert once in a while.

The headlines of smaller adverts need to be condensed

and shortened to just two or three words at most, but they still need to have the same attention grabbing affect as a bigger advert. Copy will also need to be shortened, using only the most effective and important words.

List what is important for your small advert, it should include;

● The headline.

● The name of the profession or service.

● Contact details, especially the phone number or website address.

● Any discount or voucher details.

Don't feel that you need to fill up every single millimetre of space on your advert. Sometimes white space in an advert can be just as appealing or eye stopping as a photograph.

EXAMPLES OF SMALL ADVERTS

REFLEXOLOGY

From the comfort of your own home

£5 Discount
with this advert
Valid unti 1 Dec 09

Contact
SUSAN HATFIELD

01234 567890

BACK ACHE?

Telephone
01234 567890
for an appointment

**Pro Physiotherapy
10 Exercise Lane
Sweatshire**

£5 Discount
with this advert
Valid until 1 Dec 09

IMPROVE YOUR POSTURE
in 60 minutes

The Alexander techniques demonstrated by John F Hammer could help you reduce back and limb complaints caused by poor posture.

CALL NOW FOR YOUR 60 MINUTE INTRODUCTORY ASSESSMENT

01234 567890

**John F Hammer
67 Gait Walk
Postureshire**

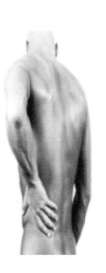

9

Utilising your Clinic

Your clinic is the most effective advert for you and your business. You have space outside and inside to educate and inform your clients about the services you offer because chances are they won't actually realise the full range of your skills. Targeting existing patients who already attend the clinic is a great way of stimulating word of mouth advertising and it's very cheap.

Whilst patients are waiting in the reception area of your clinic, they are likely to start reading the posters and leaflets your have available. Make sure they are prima-rily about you and the business, rather than having too many leaflets about other businesses or events that people have given to you to promote. Try to cover all aspects of different treatments you can provide together with people who could benefit from your services on several different posters. Have leaflets about the most common complaints you treat and don't forget to include your contact details on them, as they are likely to take it home with them. If the patient isn't interested themselves you can be sure that they know someone who will be and are likely to pass it on to them. Another place where you can inform patients about your services is in the treatment room itself, here you have an audience who cannot escape until treatment is completed which could be between 30 and 60 minutes. Put up a notice board in your treatment room with information displayed on it which stimulates conversation. This could be in the form of an interesting fact or figure, a question or information of professional advances.

Outside the clinic you have got a blank canvas to work on. Make the most of your window space and create an eye catching display or sign that draws people to look and come into the clinic. This technique works well for clothing stores and could work well for you. Changing the external appearance of your practice may require planning permission from your local authority especially if you are putting up signs or altering the fascia.

10

Directories

Whatever business you are in, it is always a good idea to get yourself listed in a telephone directory. In most cases this is the first place that people turn to when they need something and as with any other advert; you need to make sure that yours stands out from your competitors. Design your directory advert in the same way as you would an advert you place in a newspaper. It needs to have a strong headline and good copy; you may even want to include a photograph and your company logo.

The people who look in a telephone directory are not doing so to pass the time, but have made a conscious effort to find the answer to their problem. Because the reason why a person is looking in a directory and not the newspaper is different, your advert will need to be more informative. But what will make them choose you over all your competitors? It is not simply enough to have a free listing of your name and phone number. By having an advert you have already jumped the queue and are nearer to the front. You need to aim to be the first one they call. Think of your headline, it needs to be bold and clear and often your name or the name of the clinic is enough. Instead of long copy why not just have bullet points listing the conditions you treat or the types of people who can benefit from your treatment. This gives the reader a quick and clear reference list that they can scan through easily. Include your logo and contact details, if you have developed effective brand awareness already, people will instantly recognise your logo and consequently read your advert and contact the one they are most familiar with.

The Yellow Pages is still the most widely distributed and used directory available and the use of colour in this publication can definitely bring exceptional results. Because all the pages are printed on yellow paper, if you order your advert to be printed on a white background, it will instantly stand out against your competitors. It does of course cost more to have this white background, but the interest and results it generates will pay for itself time and again. If a couple of your competitors are also using a white background it will be a race to the finish based on your advert content and your reputation. Building up a strong reputation through good professional work as well as promotion will always give you the edge over someone who the potential patient has not heard of.

Inclusion of a photograph in your advert will also give you the advantage as it stands out proudly from the predominantly yellow and black page of adverts. Don't be afraid to put quite a bit of money into your Yellow Pages advert, it will always give you results. To help with the costs they will often allow you to spread the payment of your advert over ten months, interest free.

There are several other telephone directories worth getting your contact details in, as well as local handbooks or community directory's.

Don't forget about online directories as well. Yellow Pages have an online version of their big yellow book. Contact them about including your details and even a link to your website. As technology progresses you need to think more and more about getting your details onto the internet, even if you don't want to develop a website yet, you should still think about keeping your details in an electronic form so that others can search for it. More and more people are using the internet to quickly find the contact or business they need instead of rifling through the pages of a thick directory.

11

Car Signage

A very simple and cheap way of having an advert which continues to work for you day after day is to have your car made up with your business name, logo and contact details. When you compare the cost of having some professionally made vehicle decals to that of a single advert appearing in a newspaper it is a more cost effective way of advertising. Of course, you don't even have to have anything fancy, you could just have a magnetic sign which attaches to your car door.

One drawback with car signage is that you will never be able to escape the fact that everyone will know what you do, even if you are going on holiday. Everyone needs some privacy for themselves and their family and car signage will be with you wherever you are. Some people may even approach you outside of work just because you are in your 'work' car even when you may just want to be left alone.

Car signage works well with a lot of professions such as builders, plumbers and decorators but you will need to decide if the image a sign on your car gives is appropriate for a healthcare professional. Some think it degrades medical professionals but it will definitely generate new customers for you if you do decide to do it.

Two negative effects you may need to consider when using car signage, are firstly, if you are not a very good driver and others see you driving erratically, they will not be inclined to visit you as they will always associate your driving with you and your practice. Secondly, you may generate some resentment or negativity towards the type of car you drive. If it is a nice new car with your advertising on, people may think that you are too flashy and don't need their custom, but if the car is old and rusty they may think you are not very successful and consequently not a good practitioner. Peoples perceptions are peculiar, but using your car as an advert and drawing attention to it, may not always get the positive response you would hope for.

12

Post Office Advertising

Targeting other businesses to display your advert is an easy way of making the most of the people who visit them and not you. Post Offices often have display boards above the counter windows advertising local businesses. In some there is often a television displaying adverts on as well, so why not get your name in front of these people too. After all, there is not an awful lot more you can do in the queue for the Post Office than look around and if they come away with a greater awareness of you and your business, so much the better. You must remember though, that the people in the queue may not have a pen and paper with them to write your details down so make sure that your phone number or website address are easy to remember. The television display gives you the opportunity to tell a bit more about your practice than just a static printed advert. If you wish to get yourself in front of Post Office patrons, ask for the details from one of their staff. You can then supply a JPEG version of your advert or they may even design it on your behalf.

Another place where displays are available for you to put your advert, can be in a hospital waiting area or reception. This may be particularly good because the patients who visit a hospital are also likely to require your service.

Keep your eyes open for opportunities which may arise in other waiting areas, it may be worth investing in if the type of person waiting in them could also benefit from your treatment and fits your market research patient model.

13

Radio Advertising

The use of radio advertising can be quite effective especially when used in conjunction with other forms of advertising and promotion.

A radio advert is unique when compared with other formats as there are no visual stimulus or brand images to recognise. This does not mean that it doesn't work. Where as you need to pay attention when watching television or reading a newspaper or magazine, a radio can be listened to whilst doing something else, such as driving or working. Local radio will reach the relevant population surrounding your practice and chances are they will hear your advert on several occasions. Such awareness of your business then helps to increase the responses to other forms of advertising such as in the local newspaper.

Because the audience will often be doing something else when the radio is turned on, you need to make sure that your phone number and website address is memorable. That way, when they get out of the car or have their lunch break at work, they are more likely to remember what number they need to phone or better still, what your website address is. Getting people to visit your website then provides them with additional information, visually reinforces your image and branding and gives them the important contact information again.

Using a local radio station is always going to be far better for small businesses than national radio. Local community radio builds strong and loyal listeners which, over time, develop into trusting relationships. By advertising on your local radio you will be taking advantage of this relationship and the audiences' loyalty to the radio will ultimately reflect in how favourable they will react to your advert by comparison to a newspaper advert.

The presenters of radio shows also develop a personal relationship with their listeners as each day they talk about aspects of their lives as well as giving their opinions and thoughts. If you can get one of the presenters, whose voice the audience instantly recognises, to read your radio advert, it has the same instant appeal as a good headline on a written advert; it stops the audience and makes them pay attention. But this isn't where it ends, because the listeners know the presenter that advert has the same effect as a personal recommendation and that is always likely to get a better response than from an unfamiliar voice that they don't know or necessarily trust.

If you are considering advertising on the radio, a series of different but short adverts seems to get a better response than the same one repeated over and over again.

For example – you could run several adverts each depicting a person retelling the cause of their back pain and consequently the solution, which of course is going to your clinic.

By running different adverts, the audience has a greater number of things to relate to and hopefully if they see parallels between themselves and the people on the advert they will feel confident enough to contact you for your help. Variety also increases the listeners need to pay attention to your advert as they don't know which one is going to be played. You could also vary the times of the day that your advert is played. Different types of people listen to the radio at different times of the day so try to have adverts which appeal to different age groups who have different social situations.

The cost of a radio advert is also a lot less than that of a television advert, and more comparable to a run of newspaper adverts.

14

Creating an Online Presence

The use of a website is a great tool for your business. It gives more information to those who want it, serves as a permanent advert for your practice, can be found on a search engine, adds to the professional image of your practice and enhances your business as a brand.

Most health care professionals will not generally have products to sell other than their service, but information websites will still generate you money by bringing in new customers through the door.

The simplest website is one which just consists of information about you, the clinic and the services you provide. It is basically an advert for getting patients into the clinic. This type of website is quick and easy to set up and involves very little or no cost.

The first thing you need to do is to buy your Domain Name. This will be the name of the site so try and make it memorable. Usually the name of your business is used, but check whether or not the name is available first by using a Domain Checker. If you type 'web host' into a search engine it will show many results of companies that will sell you the space and software to develop a site, but they will also have a Domain Checker to see if your website name is already being used.

Typically a name ending with '.com' will cost more than '.co.uk' or others and will depend on where you purchase it from.

Even though you are purchasing your Domain Name, you are actually only leasing that name for the specified length of time. To continue using the name in the future, you will need to renew annually or biannually. You should be offered first choice at renewing the contract for your name when your current one expires, so no one else should be able to steal the name and set up a similar site under your name with what will hopefully by then be a reputable and frequently visited site.

Some web site Hosters will include a Domain Name free in their packages for hosting your site, so shop around.

Don't waste time checking to see whether or not your

Domain name is available on several different Domain Checkers. If it's not available on one, it won't be available on any of the others. Domain Checkers search the entire Internet so one checker is usually all that is required. It is only the price to register that name that will vary between sites.

Before you go 'live' with your site, it is vital that you prepare thoroughly the following;

- What text you will be including.

- How many pages the site will need to be.

- What photographs you will include.

If you can do extensive preparation before you attempt to upload the data to the Internet, it will be easier to get started, be more comprehensive and organised and look a lot more professional.

Start with the layout of the site and draw up a list of all the different pages contained in the site. Then think about how the pages will be linked to one another.

Include pages with information on different conditions and how you treat them, your contact details, a location map of your practice, biography of yourself, opening hours and a price list. You could even offer an on line booking system, so patients can choose when their appointment is. This would involve additional software to link with the computer in the reception area at your practice and may become costly.

Desirable aspects of a good website include;

- Limited or no jargon.

- Concise snappy text and information.

- Directions on why the customer needs your products.

- Follow tried and tested layouts of successful websites, such as those found as templates in hosting packages.

- Keep it simple.

- No large pictures or gimmicks.

- Restrict pop-up advertisements.

- Include a 'help' section.

Once you are happy with the structure of your site,

write out all the text for each page of your website on Microsoft Word or another universally recognised word processing programme, then all you will then need to do is 'cut and paste' the text into the site. Also, think about what photographs or graphics you want to include. Take digital photographs of your practice, your staff and different treatment methods, but make sure they are of a high quality with good resolution, especially in close up. Photos are best taken against a single coloured, neutral background. If you are going to use other people's photographs you will need their permission and you may have to pay them royalties. Where possible, use you own.

When considering the images, try to keep the size of them down. When a website is being loaded onto a potential patient's computer, the bigger the image, the longer it will take to download. The interest and attention of that patient may have evaporated if they have to wait for too long.

The more preparation you can do before you go live will make the site more organised and the transition from your computer to the internet a lot smoother. Sit on the floor with the pages of your website out in front of you with all the information and pictures on them. Only when the layout and structure works should you start to consider putting the site onto the internet for others to see. Remember that first impressions count, so don't rush into a website because if the site is not visually and factually exciting, people are not going to return, they will simply look for the sites of your competitors.

To get your site onto the web, you will need the services of a host. A good host will not only sell you your web space, but provide email facilities, manage the website, advise you on ways to improve the site, submit your site to search engines and provide performance statistics upon request. Find a host and see which package you will need to satisfy the number of pages your site consists of and shop around.

Once you have found the hosting package which is suitable for you, you have then the task of transferring all the text you have prepared for the site into the template provided by the host. Most of this can be done simply by cutting and pasting the text into the template. Many different templates will be provided for you to adapt and use as your site. They simply provide the framework on to which you can add your text and images. Although the process of getting all the relevant information of your website onto the internet may seem daunting, a lot of good hosts will help you by providing online or downloadable guides specific to their system. Print these off so that you have it in front of you. Depending on the complexity of your proposed site will dictate how long it takes for you to complete it. Save it in stages so that you can go back to it later and add to it.

Many hosts will provide you with set up wizards for all aspects of the website, all you need to do is answer the questions and supply the information. It can be time consuming uploading lots of pictures into the site, but once the initial set up is complete, any changes or additions will not take so long.

Many hosts will give you the chance to see how the site will work once it has been uploaded to the internet. Use this facility, as it will give you a good idea of how the layout, links and format will look and function before your customers do.

Even when you think that your website is complete, you may want to make continual changes and improvements to it every month. Maintaining a site which shows you and your clinic in the best possible light may need minor adjustments on a monthly basis, so make a point of going back to the site regularly.

Like any product or service that you provide, it is pointless spending money getting new equipment and making improvements or changes if your customers are not informed. The time, effort and money you have put into developing your website would all be a waste unless you tell potential patients about it.

To start with, make sure your website address is on all forms of literature, leaflets and business cards. This helps to generate good customer relations with your existing patients as well as providing them with access to your website which acts like a 24 hour representative of your business. By visiting your site, the query or information that they needed answering has been addressed quickly and without them having to contact you directly.

Any advertisements done locally in newspapers, telephone directories etc, should also have your website address clearly displayed. For potential new patients to your clinic, the website provides a lot more information than could possibly be added to the small advert in the newspaper. If patients are armed with more information they are more likely to book an appointment because they gain more confidence in you.

Search Engines are the first place that most people turn to when they are looking for something on the internet. Inputting keywords for the field you are looking for will turn up thousands of results. What you have to do is make sure that the relevant keywords and information corresponds to your site. You will also need to make sure that your site is ranked as high as possible in the search engine results.

Search Engines sift through information contained in your site from several locations including;

- *Site and Page Title* – the name of the website as well as the page names which appear at the top of the internet browser window.

- *Description* – input your website description. This is usually limited to around 200 characters and should be as specific as possible.

- *Keywords* – you can choose the keywords for your site. Often your web host will give you a section where you can input your keywords, although they may limit the volume of words or characters. It is often worth making your Home Page contain many of these words as a lot of search engines organise the relevance of your site by the Home Page text content.

- *Hyperlinks* – search engines assess the importance of a site by the number of links it has with other important websites. Don't just pick any links you can find, but choose links to other websites which are relevant to yours, such as suppliers or professional bodies. Some companies may be happy to exchange banners with you, linking both sites to each others.

It is worth sitting down and making a list of your keywords and putting some thought into your description. Put yourself in your potential customers' position; think about what you would put into a search engine if you were looking for an Osteopath or Hypnotherapist in your area. Many web hosts will automatically submit your site and keywords to many different search engines, some of which you will probably never have heard of. As long as your site is registered with the main ones it will usually be automatically included with the other various search engines. You do not need to trawl through every search engine to manually submit your site to them.

There are software packages that are available to help you optimise your website and improve your search engine rating.

Another way of improving your rating and ensuring you are on the first page of results is to do keyword advertising. This is where you purchase keywords and advertising space from a search engine to visibly increase your profile. The cost of keyword advertising can vary, but is usually based on the number of clicks on the advert which takes visitors to your site, or as a fixed fee for an entire advertising campaign.

It is also useful to register your website and clinic with business directories like www.yell.com. This is particularly useful when customers are looking for a service in a specific geographical location. Yell will charge you annually for the listing on the site as well as a set up fee.

As with many aspects of your business, you should continually review and monitor your website. Many web hosts provide analysis statistics on the performance of your site including the number of visitors, which pages they looked at and where they are located. Some will also inform you which links have been successful in bringing visitors to the site. By monitoring the habits of your customers, you can adapt and evolve your site to improve the look and content and make it more user friendly.

SECTION D

PROMOTION

Promotion

Public explanation of the benefits of a service sometimes by incentives, physical demonstrations or trials.

15

Valuing Your Customers

You may automatically think that your patients know how much you value their custom, but if they don't, it could have a negative effect on your business. There are small changes you can make to your daily practice to ensure that your patients will want to come back to you time and time again.

As a health care professional, you are placed in a very unique position in that all your patients have face to face contact with you or an associate of your business. This enables you to develop relationships with each customer, a concept which is not always possible with many businesses who may instead deal with impersonal customer orders via the phone, internet or post. Nothing develops better relationships with customers than meeting them in person.

So how can you maximise these relationships and use them to help expand your business? Without patients you have no business, you need to keep them repetitively coming back time and time again.

To understand how to satisfy your patients and meet, or better still, exceed their expectations, you need to first understand how they assess your service.

Patients judge you and your service on the following decisions:

- How good your clinical skills are.

- The convenience and facilities of your clinic.

- Feeling valued as a customer.

- Your personality.

- Price and availability of appointments.

Surprisingly, the price of your service is not necessarily the most important factor in keeping patients coming back to you. Most patients will not be put off by paying a couple of pounds more than your competitors if their perceived value of your service is greater. The saying 'You get what you pay for,' is often true. You can, of course, price your services lower than your competitors and still excel in all the other criteria suggested above, but overall, the factor which keeps the patient returning will not be the price, it will be you, as a person; your clinical skills, your personality and the feeling that they are valued by you.

You need to be able to show to your customers that you care about them as an individual person, not just as another patient on a long list of work for that day.

When a patient returns to your clinic, chances are you won't remember much about them since their last appointment two months ago, but they don't want to know that. Patients want to be treated as individuals, so make the most of your clinical notes by writing down aspects of the conversation you had with them at their last visit ready to be used at their next appointment. Write down information about what holidays they are going on, family occasions, other family members' health or what's occupying their time, e.g. training for the marathon. Armed with a refresher of what's going on in that patients' life will direct you to ask follow up questions during the course of the treatment. This makes the patient feel important, individual and gives the appearance that you have taken an interest in their life. Receptionists also need to be welcoming to the customers when they enter the building rather than wearing a blank expression and not recognising the patient. Talk to receptionists, they are the first representative of your business and as such give the vital first impression to customers of you and your business. Ask them to greet patients friendly and address them by their names.

Show patients that they are worth more to you than simply the fee you are collect from them for that treatment.

When it comes down to it, each patients visit represents money coming into the business, but the patient does not need to be made to feel that their money is all you are interested in. If they do feel that way, it's guaranteed that they will not return. A patient's visit is worth much more than just the fee for that visit, it is worth a lifetime of visiting fees as well as valuable recommendation to others for which you will receive their visiting fees. Don't view a patient's treatment as only being worth the fee they pay you, it can be worth so much more.

Make patients feel like their custom is valued and appreciated. Patient's who feel that their custom is valued and not complacently expected every time, are more likely to return time and time again. The simplest and most effective thing you can do is just say 'Thank You.' Sometimes just saying goodbye as the patient leaves and not saying thank you could leave patients feeling like they are not appreciated. After all, you probably wouldn't go back to a shop where the assistant didn't thank you, so why should your patients feel any different. Make a point of saying 'Thank you for coming,' to every patient and you may notice by comparison how frequently you had previously forgotten. Try to work to time as much as you can, people can feel very undervalued if they are kept waiting. If you are delayed, make sure the first thing you do to the patient is apologise, but ensure it sounds sincere. If patients phone you and a message is taken on your behalf, do everything you can to return the call the same day.

Patients know you are a busy person, but they still have certain expectations and deserve to feel like they are valued by you. Small adjustments could even help grow your business and retain more customers.

16

Care Packages

Your customers want reassurance that their decision to come and see you is the right one to make and won't cost them too much money. As part of your policy, why not offer a care package that gives the patient their money back if they don't benefit or are not satisfied with your service. This may seem like an extravagant way of getting customers but it's a tried and tested method that does get a lot of results. When you've gone into a supermarket and bought a bottle of shampoo I'm sure you would feel a lot more confident buying a bottle of an unknown brand as opposed to your usual brand if you could claim back your money if you were not happy with the product. The 'Money Back Guarantee' has been applied to many products and services over the years from men's electric razors to vehicle tyre replacement centres.

By publicising your care policies you are demonstrating to your market place that:

- You are confident that the service you provide is of a certain high standard.

- You must be competent in a professional capacity otherwise you would always be giving people their money back.
- The patient has nothing to loose.

- You care for your patients well being.

- You are not just interested in earning money from patients.

If you implement this policy, patients pay as they go as normal, but claim their money back after the end of treatment if they are not happy or the treatment has not worked. You need to make sure that very few people should be so unhappy with the service that they want their money back. This is helping to keep the standards high in the practice and your skills up to date and competent.

Another type of care package you could adopt is the 'Try before you buy' scheme. This is also mentioned in the 'Free Assessments' section of this book.

17

Offering Free Assessments

Like many ways to get publicity and promote your clinic to patients who don't know of you or don't know why your service would be of benefit to them, giving away something for nothing grabs the public's attention.

There are two ways of offering a free assessment;

1. As a one off promotional day.

2. As a general structure for your treatments.

Whichever one you choose to do, it will increase the volume of patients you have and raise your profile within the market place as someone who offers something unique amongst your profession.

The aim of offering free assessments is to raise awareness of you, your business and your profession. By assessing patients you should be able to tell them whether or not they would benefit from further assessment and treatment. It is not a time to provide treatment, just to ascertain whether or not it is needed. They will then need to book an appointment if treatment is required, which they will need to pay for. You have also got the opportunity to educate a client about your business. Even if they don't need it themselves, they are more likely to pass on the advice to others and in doing so, will mention you and your business.

1. As a one off promotional day

Plan your clinic and diary well in advance and allocate a day where you will only see new people for assessment. The length of time for your assessment will need to be shorter than normal so that you can get as many people into that day as possible. Keep assessments concise and to the point, but provide as much information as possible. Make sure you stock up on leaflets and business cards so that the patients you see that day go away with something that has your name and phone number on. Even if they don't need you right now, at least your number will be the one they think of ringing when they do need it. Making sure that patients leave with a leaflet is also another great way to stimulate recommendation. The patient may know someone else who may benefit from your service and can pass the leaflet to.

Because the assessments will be shorter, enrol the services of the receptionist to acquire the usual patients data, such as name, address, contact details, GP name etc. This saves you time during the assessment, but helps to satisfy accuracy in your record keeping. Another way of saving time is to provide a pre-assessment form for patients to complete themselves, containing medical history, a list of medication and any other information you may require. This form can be given to the patients when they arrive at the clinic or posted to the patient before the appointment. Completing the form at home may be easier for the patient as they will have access to their prescription to list medication easily, and have more time to think about their medical history. Don't forget to ask the patient to sign the form as consent for treatment.

Make sure that patients know that the free assessment does not include treatment before they arrive, otherwise they may leave disgruntled and create negative word of mouth advertising.

What you call the event should also be given some thought.

For example:

Podiatrists : Foot Health Awareness Day

Physiotherapists : Body Awareness Day

Reflexologists : Reflexology Advice Open Day

By giving the assessment day a name it makes it appear that it is an event that they may want to be part of rather than just a promotion of your services. As this is a one off event, you will need to inform all those that may be interested. The quickest and easiest, but unfortunately the most expensive way is to place an advert in the local newspaper. This will need to be done at least twice and up to two weeks before the event so that everyone knows.

2. AS A GENERAL STRUCTURE FOR YOUR TREATMENTS

Instead of having an incentive day for patients to come and be assessed, why not make it part of the package of treatment and give every new patient a free assessment. To recoup some of this cost you could always increase your treatment fees slightly, but overall it gives the impression that you provide a great value service. To those who don't need treatment you will be leaving them with a positive impression of you and your services which they are likely to remember as well as pass on to other potential clients. Effectively you have made the patient a walking advert for you. Positive recommendations are always the best way of getting new clients which stay with you for a long time.

Once again, the appointment time for a free assessment will need to be shorter so that it does not take up too much of your time. To save time, get all the paperwork done either before they come to the clinic or whilst they wait in the reception area of your practice.

Advertising a free assessment built into the treatment package is relatively simple. All you need to do is put up signage inside and outside of the clinic and your diary will soon start to fill up. You may want to put an advert in the local newspaper to get the ball rolling but once the word has spread, any additional newspaper adverts will not be required.

Giving a free assessment as part of your package of treatment works well for many other professions, including builders and contractors, double glazing and conservatory salesmen. The 'try before you buy' system works well because it gives the client a certain sense of reassurance that it won't cost them anything, even if they don't feel that it is right for them. To you, it will mean that you will have to maintain the very highest standards and skills, otherwise you will soon lose money and your business will run at a loss due to the lack of treatments you will be physically paid for.

To grow at a relatively quick rate and with a positive reputation within your local community, you will need to invest some time, money and effort in putting yourself across to your market place. If you don't your business could fail or develop so slowly that it will run out of money even if you are a wonderful clinician.

18

Open Days

By having an open day, you are inviting anyone who may be interested in your services to simply visit the premises, see if they like what they see, feel comfortable with the surroundings and ask you questions. This is an effective way of developing trust between yourself and the patients, especially those who haven't been to you before, and putting their mind at ease. Some people can be quite nervous or hesitant about trying something new and by visiting an open clinic, they are under no pressure or obligation to use you in the future.

Your main objective of hosting an open day is to impress the patient by your clean and professional clinic, then make them realise why they could benefit from attending for treatment. Like a lot of promotion, you are going to be imparting advice and knowledge to your patients so that they become educated and make an informed decision about their health and where they go to obtain treatment.

If you work in a clinic where there are many different health professionals, an open day can be an excellent way of getting overall promotion for each practitioner in one go. There may be people who attend the open day out of curiosity for one profession but end up booking appointments for several different practitioners. Make sure that all of the practitioners are present at the open day. It is just as important for people to chat and get to know you as it is for them to experience the clinic and its facilities. You are going to build up a loyal customer base if you allow them to get to know you, and this type of customer will be the sort who repeatedly uses you and your practice because they've taken the time and effort to personally develop a relationship with you. If this pleasant interaction is reciprocated by you, the patient is always more likely to choose you over a stranger when they need treatment. They are also much more likely to recommend you to their friends because they will talk about you with such fondness. It goes without saying that you should always act in a professional and proper manner, but that doesn't mean you cannot be friendly.

Make the open day a 'bit of an occasion.' Serve drinks

and snacks so that people will stop and talk to you, your colleagues as well as other patients for longer. The more they feel comfortable and part of the clinic, the happier they will feel about booking an appointment. Have some background music on, so that the situation does not feel too clinical. If it is an actual opening day celebration, why not ask someone of local importance to come and cut the ribbon, chances are the press will also turn up and write a feature on the practice and you will gain some valuable advertising for the event. Don't forget to have plenty of leaflets and information to hand out to everyone and as an incentive for that day, some discount vouchers to be used for treatment when they book an appointment.

Another type of open day is one aimed at other health care practitioners. Although they are not as likely to book an appointment with you as you would get in an open day for the general public, you will be allowing other professionals to get to know you and understand more fully what it is you do, where you work, what facilities you have and what conditions you treat. By making them more aware of you they are more inclined to refer their patients to you for treatment. Building positive relationships with other professions is vital for your practice to develop a good reputation within your local community and eventually you will find that most of your new patients will come via patient and professional recommendations and the need to embark on additional advertising and promotion will not be required.

19

Events and Demonstrations

If the general public can see what you do, maybe try it out for free and become more educated in the benefits of your treatment, they are much more likely to use you and your clinic. Building up an awareness of your business can be quite simply done by attending local events, fetes or open days and physically demonstrating your service. Plan ahead and be selective on which events you will be attending, after all you will be there for the whole day and the last thing you want is to be sat there with nothing to do. Keep an eye on the events taking place locally to you in your local newspaper, directory or handbook. There is no point doing a demonstration in an area which is miles away from your clinic, people will not travel to you for an appointment. Often organised events will be arranged through a professional company who may be responsible for several in the area, contact them for information of forthcoming events and costs. It may be good to contact your local district council and schools who may also arrange occasional events at various locations.

On the day of the event take some basic equipment as well as a couple of friends or family members who can pose as members of the public and be the first to volunteer to try you out. This acts as a stimulus for others to try as no one usually likes to be the first. You can structure your day however you want to, but the main aim is to see as many people as possible so that you are bringing an awareness of your practice to them. It is better to provide a shortened treatment so that there is something for others to see as well as keeping the queue moving. If it is just assessments you provide, it could mainly be observed as being talking between yourself and your patient and will not inspire others to book or join the queue for their trial. You could have a sheet of paper for people to add their names to at allotted times, this way you are keeping a steady momentum of work flowing and patients have a choice. Alternatively you could simply have a queue system, however people may be put off with having to wait or stand for long periods of time. Allotted times tend to work better, as it also gives people the chance to look around the rest of the event whilst waiting for you. If you work in a multidisciplinary practice, take someone else with you to work along side you. Having more than one practitioner works well because a husband and wife or two friends can book at the same time so they don't become separated.

When appearing in public, make sure you have plenty of information about yourself and the clinic so that the public have something to take away with them to look at later. As with other forms of promotion, providing some money off vouchers is a certain way of getting an immediate response, but be careful about how many you supply as some people may take more than one. In this case you would have to specify only one per person and when they did use it in the clinic you would have to make a note, so they cannot repeat the discount at a later stage. To encourage people to try your service whilst you are at the event, you could always specify that only those who try you will receive a discount voucher.

As well as local events, you could participate in those slightly further a field, as long as you can get some local press coverage of yourself being at the event. Volunteering for work at events such as the London Marathon, Great North Run, Commonwealth Games, Football and Cricket clubs, Homeless centres etc, will all give you some valuable promotion. You will not need to pay for working at these events as you are providing a service for free. Tell your local newspaper what you are doing and they may want to write an article about you.

20

Talks and Presentations

A simple way of gaining new patients as well as making your presence known in your local community is to give free talks. But it is important not to waste you time talking to the wrong groups of people. By under-taking market research you should have established a sound understanding of your potential customers and where they may frequent as well as which clubs or groups they belong to.

The easiest and quickest ways to find out the location and timetable for these meetings may include;

- Talking to existing patients and gaining the contact details for the organiser or manager.

- Visiting the local library. They will hold information on all sorts of local groups.

- Local and community newspapers. Some

will have listings of which groups are meeting each month. Don't worry if you've missed the current date, at least you have the contact information.

- Internet. A lot of groups may have their own website, but if not they may be part of a larger 'parent' group whose site may hold local group information.

- For larger organisations such as Diabetes UK, Arthritic Research Council, Woman's Institute etc contact their main office (found on the internet) and they will be able to put you in touch with a local representative.

- Visit existing businesses which provide services to people who may be relevant to your business, such as Gymnasiums, Age Concern or GP surgeries.

- If you have a village or community hall, they may hold information on relevant groups, some of which may even use the hall to hold their meetings in.

Once you have found gatherings of people who fit your typical patient model you will need to write some talks to take to them. Some talks you will be able to reuse for different groups, whereas others may just need adjusting slightly to make them more applicable. Either way you will probably build up a stock of about 3 different talks, parts of which will be repeated in all of them.

Contact the groups and see if they would be interested in having you talk to their members. Meeting groups often get booked up ahead, especially if they only get together once a month so don't be surprised if the date they offer you is a few months ahead. In some ways this is good; it means you won't need to rush the preparation for your talk. Unfortunately, it also means there is a delay in capitalising on the interest in your business a talk will generate.

Take your time when writing your talk and when reviewing what you have written, try to look at it from the perspective of your audience. If you wander off the track and it becomes irrelevant to your audience, they will become bored and uninterested in you, your profession and your business.

When writing the talk try to think of the visual aids that you can incorporate into it. People take in a lot more information when they can see things rather than just listen to a voice. If possible, try to get some audience participation and get them involved with the subject you are talking about. Demonstrating something on a member of the audience makes the talk much more fun for them as it does for you. The key thing you need to remember is that you want these people to use your business. Although you are there to educate and inform them, you need to get them to remember you, use you and recommend you. If they don't, then your talk will have been a waste of your time.

As well as making your talk interesting, you need to be able to link it or direct it in such a way that you are also able to talk to the audience about your practice and the service you provide. Don't make this too obvious or it will just appear to be a sales pitch, which of course it is, but they don't need to know that. Just by being at the meeting and talking to them, the audience will automatically link you with your profession. By listening to you they will hopefully understand the relevance your profession has to them and by informing them of the location and name of your practice it will prompt them to use you.

Brand awareness is a tool which will play an important part in your talk. On literature, pictures, computer presentations or slides, make sure your logo is clearly displayed. It is putting your business in front of the audience without them realising it.

Some of your audience will want more information from you so be prepared for questions at the end, some of which could be personal questions about their own health and how you could help them. Try not to give too much away, talk to them about possible solutions or treatments and how they may help, but advise them to come to the clinic for a more in depth consultation. Take with you plenty of leaflets about the clinic and the services you provide. Discount vouchers are always a good way to prompt people into the clinic. Take some with you, but make sure they are date sensitive, i.e. don't let them use the voucher indefinitely. Make the voucher expire within 3-4 weeks after the talk so that people are prompted to use them soon after the talk whilst it is still fresh in their minds.

Before the day of the talk comes, practice a few times doing your talk in front of family or friends or in front of the mirror. Try to make yourself familiar with your talk so that you are not constantly looking down at the sheet of paper you are reading from. The more familiar you are with the talk the less you will need to look at your papers except as a cue which makes your presentation much better.

When the talk comes along, arrive early to get yourself prepared and familiar with your surroundings. It can be quite daunting talking to 10, 20 or 30 people, so try to relax yourself by taking deep breaths and sitting calmly before the talk. If it helps, try to visualise yourself giving the talk to a happy and interested audience and the presentation going perfectly. Remember that the audience will only ask you questions on a subject you know about; your job, so you shouldn't have trouble answering them.

21

Testimonials

The one important thing that will make new patients hesitate about coming to see you or not is fear of the unknown. They don't know what you are like or whether your treatment will be right for them. They won't know if you are any good at your job or if they want to part with their hard earned money to you.

The easiest way to calm the potential patients' fears is to tell them what the experience will be like, but they are more likely to believe someone who has been to you before, rather than you telling them. Unfortunately, they may not know anyone who has already been to you, so their fears remain.

A testimonial, where patients write down their opinion or recommendation of their experience for others to read, can be included on all your literature and adverts as well as your website. This acts as a personal recommendation to others, even though it is from someone the reader of the leaflet does not know.

To obtain a testimonial you will first need to ask existing patients to write down their opinion of the treatment and service they receive from your practice. Make them aware that their opinion could be used on your promotional material. It may be a good idea to write this down and get the patient to sign it if they agree. Some patients may be happy to give you their opinion for you to use, but may themselves prefer some anonymity. If this is the case you can simply use "speech marks" to specify that it is a quote or write underneath the title and first letter of their name, such as 'Mr F. Ashford, Kent.'

Another way to obtain a testimonial is to gain permission to use quotes from letters that grateful patients have already sent to you.

There are a couple of good side effects that getting existing patients to write down their opinions has on your business. Firstly, it highlights to you, what your business is doing well and what areas could perhaps do with some further attention. This sort of feedback is valuable to businesses but so often overlooked. Getting to know your patients and what they like and dislike can help to grow your business a lot quicker.

Secondly, by getting patients to think about what they like about the treatment at your practice, helps them to formulate a clearer picture in their mind. When they are talking to their friends about you, they are more likely to give a better formulated description and consequently a better recommendation. As was written earlier, patients who currently don't use you are much more likely to if you come recommended by someone who has already tried you.

Testimonials are simple and cheap, but more effective than you first may think.

22

Promoting Your Practice with Literature

When considering the range of conditions that you are qualified to treat, a lot of patients will be unaware of how comprehensive a service you can actually provide. For some problems, they would not even consider that their discomfort or pain would come under your remit, looking instead for treatment from other professionals or simply going down the surgical route without exploring all the other alternatives. If you have good relations with other health professionals, they may still refer these patients directly to you, for your input. But if you don't, or they are still being developed, how are you going to let patients know the scope of what you actually do treat?

You could of course, put up a sign in your clinic listing all the skills or services you provide, however, you have to consider the available space and the use of jargon which patients may not understand. Another, more effective way is to make the means available for patients to almost self diagnose their problem and thereby subtly direct themselves into your clinic. This can be done with information booklets.

If a patient picks up a leaflet, they can identify their problem using easy text and illustrations, read what they should do about it at home, and see that they need to consult you for your opinion.

EXAMPLE

Mrs Brown is sitting in the waiting area of a multi disciplinary clinic waiting to see the Physiotherapist. Whilst waiting, she is naturally looking around the room as well as scanning the literature available. She notices a booklet call 'Foot and Leg Problems' and picks it up. Mrs Brown has been having some problems with her knees lately, after she'd started taking up hiking. At first she dismissed the pains, but as they didn't get better she went to see the Physiotherapist.

On opening the booklet, the first line she reads is about how walking and foot position could cause problems in the feet, ankles, knees and hips. She has instantly become aware of a new possibility to what could be causing her knee pain. Looking at a chart within the booklet, she identifies the location of her pain, reads about its relation to foot posture and becomes more knowledgeable about her problem. Now that Mrs Brown knows what may be causing her knee problem she is then informed of the solution, including exercise, suitable footwear and an insole or orthotic. With your contact details on the booklet you are therefore the solution to where to obtain the insole or orthotic. By understanding more about her problem, Mrs Brown has looked at a possible diagnosis and treatment that she hadn't previously been aware of and so has self referred herself to you.

Because Mrs Brown has learnt something new, she is also more likely to talk to her friends about it and thereby educate them and recommend you in the process.

Another great reason to have booklets in your clinic is so that patients can take the information home with them and refer to at a later stage or give to friends or family who may also have problems.

Brief informative 3 fold leaflets can be simply made on your home computer and printed out with your name, address and contact details on. A more comprehensive booklet can be designed and written, then produced at a local printer. Although you will have to pay for each booklet, you will find that the number of patients it brings to you will be higher than comparable spending on a newspaper advertisement.

Booklets should be left at key locations where patients are likely to visit such as your clinic waiting area, GP waiting areas, Age Concern reception areas or Gymnasium reception areas for example.

Another easy promotional piece of literature for professions which deal with Sports men and women could be a concertinaed leaflet with concise reference information on exercises or specific sports related injuries, for Athletes to keep in their sports bag. If, or when, an injury occurs they have a quick guide to the problem and once again, a direct link to you. Back this piece of literature up with your phone number and offer sports clubs free telephone advice. You are then seen as an important team member of the club and as such referrals will be made to your clinic.

There are many different ways for all types of health care professionals to develop series of booklets and leaflets for patients to read and absorb. Try to make them useful so that they are kept for longer and not simply discarded when they have been read.

23

Newsletters

Over time you will gradually develop an extensive database of names and addresses of people who, at some stage, have been associated or in contact with your business. This database may include:

- Existing patients.

- People who have enquired about your services.

- People who have entered your competitions.

- Those who have attended open days.

- Those you have given a talk to.

This database is very valuable, because you have in your possession an actual list of people who your market research was directing you towards. Although not every one in the database will have used your service or received treatment from you, they are all aware of you, your skills and knowledge and the service they are likely to receive from your practice. The average person often puts off doing something until they feel they really need to, so why not give them a gentle reminder, or prompt, that they need you right now.

Design a newsletter on your computer which covers at least one side of an A4 sheet. Include information in the newsletter which is relevant to your patients such as;

- New services that you are qualified to provide and how that will benefit patients.

- Developments in the practice building which provide improved facilities.

- Changes to staff.

- What new equipment you have and why it is relevant to patient care.

- Any changes in opening times.

- Information on national or professional requirements which affect your patients.

When writing the newsletter, keep the information short, concise and clear so that it is easy to read and patients can simply pick out what is relevant to them. Include some pictures to improve the overall appearance and including facts, figures and statistics are also good to put in as it inspires interest.

Don't forget to include your business name, address and telephone details so that they know who it is from. To really get a quick response to your newsletter you could include a discount voucher on the accompanying letter. This will generate immediate interest in the letter as it is less likely to be scan read, identified as junk mail and disposed of. If they can see that the letter has some monetary value they are more likely to read it.

The cost of producing a newsletter once or twice a year is merely the cost of your time when writing it and the price of a stamp, but you are likely to get a number of people responding to it and thereby recouping the cost of the promotion.

Instead of just producing an A4 printed sheet, why not look at doing something of a better quality? You could develop an A5 booklet with lots more information and promotion about you and your profession, but also include adverts for local businesses and shops which your market may also use and approach them with your idea. Work out the cost of an advert in your booklet by taking into account printing and production costs and delivery, then adding on a profit for yourself and don't forget the tax you will have to pay. Try to keep it a reasonable fee as you are more likely to get a positive response from other businesses. Make sure that you are clear on the type of person you are mailing the booklet to so that they can appreciate the relevance your database also has to their own business. Not only will you gain some business from customers coming back to you, you will also have your promotion paid for by the sale of other businesses advertising.

24

Gift Vouchers

Selling gift vouchers in your clinic is an easy way to stimulate positive recommendations from your existing patients and gain new ones.

If a patient buys a gift voucher from you, the likelihood is that they are purchasing it for someone else rather than for themselves. By the act of giving the voucher to their friend or relative they are subconsciously endorsing you, your treatment and your practice. This is positive recommendation or word of mouth advertising and it is totally free.

The only thing you will need to pay for when producing gift vouchers is the printing of the vouchers themselves. However, this need not be expensive. You can easily print a voucher from your home computer on some good quality paper and place them inside a gift card or envelope.

The voucher will need to have details of your practice and where they can redeem it, together with the value of the voucher. It is also a good idea to include a small concise list of the treatments, services or conditions that you treat on the front of the voucher. Make sure it is clear on the voucher that it cannot be redeemed at any other practice or clinic other than yours. You can put an expiry date on the voucher as well if you wish to prompt the new patient into the clinic within the specified time limit.

If you have a multipractitioner clinic, you could offer vouchers which are generic for anything in your practice including the services and products, but to truly gain a new patient it would be more effective to only provide the vouchers for treatment. This really gets the patient to experience your care and attention and hopefully become a regular patient.

Of course, some people when they receive a voucher may not even use it, or may loose it. If this occurs then you have financially gained from the purchase of the voucher without actually having done anything.

Gift vouchers are a great way of gaining free promotion via your existing patients without too much effort. The only draw back is the promotion that the vouchers bring can be quite slow.

25

Leafleting

Leafleting an area of homes is a very cheap and quick way of generating a few new patients. All you need to do is print off some leaflets on your computer and spend some time walking around a selected area and placing them through each letter box. You can either blanket leaflet a whole area of your neighbourhood or listen to your existing patients who will give you clues about which areas have a high concentration of your target audience.

However, this method of trying to gain new patients has two problems. The first being the very poor response rate. For every thousand leaflets you put through a door, you may literally get 1 or 2 new people walking through yours. The usual response to junk mail from most households is to put it straight in the box for recycling. Only a handful of people will actually take the time to read your leaflet and of those, even less will actually want or need your services.

The second problem is whether or not random leafleting is a professional way to promote yourself. Think of the image it portrays to the potential patient when they see your leaflet coming through the door unannounced. To some it may seem a bit desperate. Check with your professional body, they may have guidelines or advice for leafleting and may not actively recommend their members to participate in such a form of promotion.

If you do decide to leaflet for new patients then you will probably gain a few, but your brand image and practice values may not be as prominent or clear as you may have developed through other adverts or promotional schemes. There are many other types of promotion you can try which involve less walking and gain you many more patients without degrading your reputation or image.

26

Running a Competition

Running a competition is an easy way of building up a database of people who are interested in your service. When there is something on offer at a reduced rate, or totally free of charge, most people find it very hard to resist, especially if it is in a service or business that they would like to experience.

Think about your business, what could you give away that would be useful and tempting to customers. You might want to think about giving away:

- A free treatment.

- A package of products you sell.

- Vouchers to be spent in your clinic.

Whatever it is, it has to be bigger than just a £5 discount

or a tube of cream, but it is counter productive making it too big. The prize has to be relevant to your business and preferably involves them experiencing the service you provide. Put yourself in the shoes of your customers; would you be tempted by your prize? Like a lot of ways to promote your business it will involve a small financial cost, but that cost will seem insignificant when you compare it to the overall benefit it will have on your business.

Once you have an idea on the final prize of the competition, you need to start thinking about the structure of the competition. Your main objective is to acquire the names and addresses of people in the marketplace who are interested in your business. To do this people will need to submit their details to enter the competition via email, the postal service or pre-printed cards. Depending on how you want to advertise the competition will vary the way entries are submitted.

- **Placing an advert in a local newspaper or handbook**. Any advert you choose to do in newspapers will always tend to be quite expensive. Some areas produce a local handbook for the area and advertising in that may cost slightly less, but will it have the same impact or circulation as an advert in the newspaper? If you do decide to place an advert in either of these mediums you will need to make it stand out from those around it. For those entering the competition, you can add the phone number of your clinic or email address for people to leave their name and address on.

- **Other peoples' businesses**. You could always leave a poster inside the premises of other businesses and shops. This is a lot cheaper to do but the response you get will be much lower. This is mainly because people will forget the contact details before they get home or loose interest because the effort to enter the competition is too great. Instead of putting a poster up, why not consider leaving a small container with a letter box type hole for customers to put their details in. This box can then be collected by you at the end of the competition. Don't make the box too big otherwise it may alienate the owner of the business you are leaving it in and they may not want to allow it space. You will also need a supply of cards for people to write on. This method of getting participation in your competition is certainly very cheap but you will rely on the goodwill of other

businesses in displaying your information.
When deciding on which businesses to leave
your competition details in, make sure it is
relevant to your market and fits the model
for your average patient.

- **Prepaid cards**. In a similar way to the last
  option, you could get some postage paid
  cards made up with details of the
  competition and space for the entrant to
  write their name and address on. As these
  take up less room on a shelf or table, other
  businesses are more likely to be cooperative.
  It becomes a little bit more expensive but
  saves you time, as you will not need to
  collect the cards at the end.

Before you decide on where to advertise your competition, don't forget to announce on the advert when the competition will end. Once it has ended and you have accumulated all the entrants you will then need to process all the data you have on the cards. The first thing you need to do is to randomly pick a winner. This can be simply done by putting the all of the names into a hat and picking one out. The winner will then need to be informed that they have won. Send them a letter together with details of the prize they have won and how they can claim it. If you can get the winner to come into your clinic to claim their prize you can then use the event as another promotional piece of advertising. Invite the local newspaper to come and write an article on the competition, the winner and your clinic. A lot of the time the article will be free but they may request you have an advert in the same issue. Try to get a photograph of your winner with you or in the practice, it will be useful for other promotional material.

Even though there is only one winner, you can still make use of the other names and addresses you have acquired. Send each person who entered a letter explaining that they have not been the winner, but thank them for entering. Remember to include a leaflet to give them more information about the clinic and a discount voucher with your compliments. This will generate additional interest in your practice and you will have an influx of new customers.

Running a competition increases your profile within your local community. You are given a golden opportunity to talk directly to people who have shown an interest in your business. Even those who do not win the competition will not be disappointed and you are seen as a genuine, kind and caring professional. This can only have a positive affect on your business, not only now but in the future too. A word of warning; do not run competitions too frequently otherwise it could start to have an adverse effect on your customers.

The database of names and addresses can be stored and retrieved when you need to publicise something. If you have a new development, expansion plans or new staff you can send information to your list of people and start stimulating additional interest.

27

Targeting Other Peoples' Businessses

Not only should you take full advantage of your own premises, but you should try to get your name in front of potential clients when they visit other peoples businesses too.

If you have done your market research effectively, you should have an understanding of your typical client and the type of group your business is relevant to. This should also give you an idea of which other businesses they would typically visit, possibly including Gymnasiums, Shoe Shops, Other Health Professionals, Age Concern, Leisure Centres etc. Think carefully about other businesses which your patients may visit. Rather than blanket advertising everywhere, concentrate on places of real significance and relevance, any money spent on advertising there is much more likely to be recouped.

Once you have come up with a list of relevant types of businesses or shops, start to make it more detailed by going though your local phone directory and find names and addresses. When you are satisfied with the list you will need to put together your advertising literature.

This can consist of;

- A poster. Make up two different size posters in A4 and A3 size. Glossy paper looks best for posters and helps to maintain the durability of them, but these would need to be printed professionally. If you want to produce an A4 poster on your computer you can make it stand out by framing it in a simple black frame. The only disadvantage of this is that the other business may not be happy with you putting nails or screws into their walls. When designing a poster follow the guidelines included in this book on designing an advert, the same applies even though it's a bigger canvas.

- Business Cards. Cards provide a handy form of advertising which can be easily placed in a pocket or wallet. Other businesses may not be too happy though if your business cards begin to spread across their work surfaces or get knocked onto the floor for them to tidy up. They will soon become annoyed by your cards and may dispose of them. If you are going to leave business cards, supply them in a container. You can purchase handy frosted plastic business card boxes from stationery suppliers very cheaply. Do not supply the lid to the box though, so that your cards will always be on display.

- Practice leaflets. If you've caught the eye of a potential customer, their initial response will be to gain more information. A leaflet should provide further information about you, your practice, the services you provide, your opening hours and costs. You can easily and cheaply print some A4 folded leaflets on your computer, but make sure that it looks professional, which also means folding it in the right place and square to the rest of the sheet of paper, so don't rush it. It is also a good idea not to photocopy your leaflet as the print quality is often not as good and slowly becomes more and more off centre. The display of leaflets is also very important. If they are scattered on the top of a table or shelf, there is less potential for them to catch the eye of the potential customer. It is much better if they can be displayed upright. Purchase a leaflet stand from a stationery stockist and put in enough leaflets to half fill it. If the leaflets have been put together in a rush they will not sit square inside the stand and will look untidy. Do not overfill the stand otherwise they may be difficult for people to remove or an excess of leaflets may overspill onto the floor. Make the stand more personal and more professional by placing an adhesive label with the business name and logo onto the clear plastic front. Improve the awareness of your business at every opportunity. Even the people who don't want a leaflet will begin to recognise your logo and associate you with your profession.

- Promotional offers. Nothing gets a response from people than the feeling that they are getting something cheaper than they normally would. There are many ways to have promotional offers, but the best way is money off vouchers. It may seem that you are giving away some of your hard earned profit, but you are getting someone through the door who might otherwise not have

done and you are inviting them to
experience your practice and service. If you
do a good job, they are likely to return to
you at some stage and recommend you to
their friends too. For the sake of a one off
small discount you have gained promotion,
advertising, loyalty and word of mouth
which are worth many times more than the
original voucher. Again you can use your
home computer to print off some vouchers
that can look just as professional as those
from a printer. Make vouchers bigger than
business cards, the size of a postcard works
well. Use a paper which is as thick as your
printer can take, glossy photo paper looks
professional. Your voucher should not just
have the value of the discount, but should
also have a brief bit of information on what
services are available at your clinic. With
any literature you are producing yourself,
make it visually attractive, using colour
where possible. Don't just print out a load of
text like a word processor document, but
break it up into bullet points, use a
professional looking font of different sizes
but limit it to only one or two types of font,
include pictures, but not too many and don't
forget the most important thing; your name,

logo, address and phone number.

When you have developed a series of advertising literature that you are happy with you need to start
approaching the businesses on your list. It is always
best to personally go into the business or shop and ask
them face to face whether they would be happy
displaying some of your literature. Ask to talk to the
manager or person in charge. A lot will refuse to
display anything and some may only be happy taking
certain things that will fit in with their displays. One
way to encourage the owners is to offer them a free
treatment as a way of thanking them for their coopera-
tion. They are then more likely to recommend your
services to their customers and you have gained a new
client.

28

Become a Source of Advice

If you can become a source of information and advice your esteem in the local community will become quite elevated. New patients will come to you simply because of your apparent position of authority in your profession. You will become the unauthorised voice in your local community to whom patients will look to first before anyone else.

There are several ways that you can provide advice for free, but that does not mean that you are going to be out of pocket. A lot of promotion involves a little bit of effort and time, and this is also the case here, but the rewards can often be better than a written advert in a newspaper and often the affects of the promotion can have a lot more benefit in the long term too.

Contact your local radio station and see if they would be interested in you coming into the station to take part in a phone-in for their listeners. Callers could phone in with questions and you can provide general advice about different conditions and how they can be treated. Keep your advice informative and useful but make sure that you keep the audience wanting to find out more, and then you tell them where they can get it from, i.e. your practice or website.

But why would a radio station want or need you to give their listeners information? How do you know it would be relevant to them? Do some research on the station and its listeners and couple that with the information you have gained from your own market research for your practice. Present to the radio controller or producer, a business like approach to your proposition. Give them the facts and figures why their listeners would benefit from hearing from you. Try to get the radio interview to correspond with a national awareness week associated with your profession. This gives it a bit more credibility and the radio station is more likely to use you for it as you have brought it to their attention and they won't want to be left out.

Another way of providing information whilst promoting yourself is by writing a feature or column for your local newspaper. Each month you could provide a written piece of information on a certain common condition which you treat, talk about its causes and highlight the treatment. An article in a newspaper is usually between 500 and 2000 words, but once you've approached the Editor, they may specify a length to fit in with their layout. It may also be more beneficial to try and write something topical or applicable to recent news or local issues so that is does not appear to be such an obvious plug for you and your clinic.

When you have a topic which is suitable to write about, beneficial for you, and informative for the newspaper and its readers, you need to contact the Editor. Explain to him in a business like manner about the article you would like to put forward and why it is in the interest of the readers for the newspaper to publish it. The Editor may not be interested but if he is, he will probably tell you what format he would like it to take. Ask for a deadline, which you must meet at all costs, and get the article written the way the Editor wants. If he doesn't approve it, there is no way it will get into the newspaper, so try to make the article right first time. Listen carefully to what he wants.

If the Editor is unsure whether to take an article from you because you are not known and the relevance may be unclear, he may ask you for a synopsis. You could always suggest yourself that you send in a synopsis if you feel the Editor is undecided. A synopsis is about 50-100 words long, explains the relevant points of the article as well as a brief explanation of what qualifies you to write authoritatively on the subject. If the Editor likes your synopsis and you have given him confidence in your own abilities he may then ask you for your article.

Columns in newspapers generally take the form of a question and answer type of format such as an 'agony aunt' page in a magazine. At least with this sort of feature you are getting direct feedback from your audience on what it actually is that they want information and help with.

Whether you are writing for a newspaper or talking on the radio, you need to make sure that the subject you are talking about is interesting and factual. Include statistics in your article if you have accurate and proven ones, which you have the source for. This makes your article fascinating and attention grabbing.

Other ways you could provide your service for free could include a free advice phone number for Sports Clubs, Gymnasiums, Schools, Age Concern, Women's Groups, Police Force, Fire Brigade, Ministry of Defence etc. Keep a separate phone line that deals purely with advice. Don't choose too many groups to provide this advice to, otherwise you will spend most of your time answering the phone, just concentrate on one or two groups who would benefit the most from your help.

Most of the time your advice will probably involve them attending the clinic for treatment, which is what you obviously need to keep the business running. If you have an informative website you could also advise them to look there for further information. Whatever happens, even if only 50% of the people who contact you need treatment, you are going to get positive exposure within your community and this can only have an expanding influence for your business.